Human Growth after Birth

DAVID SINCLAIR

Emeritus Professor of Anatomy,
University of Western Australia
Formerly Regius Professor of Anatomy,
University of Aberdeen

PETER DANGERFIELD

University of Liverpool,
New Medical School,
Liverpool

SIXTH EDITION

OXFORD   NEW YORK   TOKYO
OXFORD UNIVERSITY PRESS
1998

Oxford University Press, Great Clarendon Street, Oxford OX2 6DP
Oxford New York
Athens Auckland Bangkok Bogota Buenos Aires Calcutta
Cape Town Chennai Dar es Salaam Delhi Florence Hong Kong Istanbul
Karachi Kuala Lumpur Madrid Melbourne Mexico City Mumbai
Nairobi Paris São Paolo Singapore Taipei Tokyo Toronto Warsaw
and associated companies in
Berlin Ibadan

Oxford is a registered trade mark of Oxford University Press

Published in the United States
by Oxford University Press Inc., New York

A catalogue record for this book is available from the British Library

Library of Congress Cataloging in Publication Data
Sinclair, David Cecil.
Human growth after birth / David Sinclair, Peter Dangerfield.—6th ed.
Includes bibliographical references (p. 239).
1. Human growth.   I. Dangerfield, Peter.   II. Title.
QP84.S46   1998   612.6—dc21   98-18135

ISBN 0 19 262905 0 (Pbk)

Typeset by Technical Typesetting Ireland
Printed in Great Britain by Biddles Ltd., Guildford and King's Lynn

OXFORD MEDICAL PUBLICATIONS

Human Growth after Birth

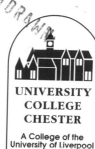
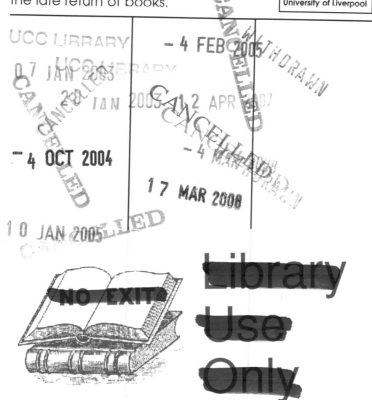

Preface to the sixth edition

In accepting the challenge of revising the text of this book, which formed the background to my own knowledge of growth as a medical student, I was also very much aware of its easy to approach readability which undoubtedly contributed to its success. To maintain this formula was not an easy task as the continual temptation was to recast text and introduce complex ideas and concepts into the new edition, the first for 9 years. In the intervening years discoveries have continued to be made in molecular biology which have led to the identification and synthesis of many new growth promoting agents and hormones. The genes controlling some of these agents have been identified and our knowledge of the internal structure and workings of the growing cell has increased. Furthermore, the explosion of medical knowledge linked to the genetics of cancer and the biological unravelling of the human genome continue to change our perception of both the normal and abnormal state of the growing and mature human body.

I have therefore introduced some of these ideas into the text, which I hope maintain and build upon the original concept of the book as devised by David Sinclair. His support has proven invaluable although he is adamant that I state that he had no hand in the revisions! A new chapter has been introduced which adds comments about the effects of the environment on growth and the final chapter on the effects of ageing has been modified to take account of new definitions and hypotheses. Several new illustrations have been employed and several short boxes within the text which address specific topics have been introduced. Inevitably this has led to a further increase in length of the book but, at all stages, I have attempted to maintain the readability of a general text which should continue to be useful to students of medicine and related health care specialities as well as those taking courses in human biology in both secondary and tertiary education.

Liverpool   PHD
1998

Contents

1 Nature of growth

Growth is a word, a term, a notion, covering a variety of diverse and complex phenomena
Paul Weiss

Definition

Growth as a concept is familiar to us all. As living organisms, we have all grown, and think we can speak from the experience. Parents set great store on seeing how their children are growing, and many readers may well remember being stood up against a convenient door or wall to be measured by their mothers. Nevertheless, not many parents understand the biological processes taking place in the child they are measuring which are causing it to grow bigger, or how their own child's progress can be related to that of other children.

The fact that growth is such a commonplace experience affecting all living things has perhaps hindered proper investigation of the factors involved, and it is only within the last 20 years or so that scientists have begun to understand the complex processes involved.

Growth can be defined as: 'The progressive development of a living being or any of its parts from its earliest stage to maturity, including the attendant increases in size'.

Similarly, the definition of 'development' is 'The series of changes by which the individual embryo becomes a mature organism'.

These definitions tell us a great deal.

First, note that growth is not just the addition of material to achieve an increase in size but a whole series of events and changes. These changes include alterations in the form of the body as a whole as well as in the form of its individual organs and systems and the specialization of various parts of the body to perform different functions. Materials such as bone and fat are added, but other material is actually subtracted. For example, the thymus gland, which is large and prominent up to about age 6 years, gradually degenerates until in the adult it has little remaining function. In the same way, vascular channels which were needed by the circulation of blood in the embryo but serve no useful purpose after birth become converted into fibrous functionless vestiges.

Growth thus includes the incidental destruction and death of cell and tissues. Such destruction is sometimes said to be 'programmed', as it forms part of the programme of normal growth. It may occur as early in development as the blastocyst stage.

Growth may also involve substitution, for example, when cartilage is converted into bone, or when the permanent teeth replace the milk teeth. Less drastic are alterations and modifications in the shape of the bony skeleton as a result of the secondary sex changes.

Similar modifications take place on the microscopic scale: for example, the cells through which filtration takes place in the kidney are cubical at birth, but later become flattened to facilitate the passage of material through them.

Secondly, the dictionary definitions distinguish between the growth of the whole 'living being' and the growth of its parts, and this is important because not all parts of the body grow at the same rate. Nor do they all stop growing simultaneously. Furthermore, growth of one part may be controlled by the activity of another (such as the endocrine system), and the degree of control will depend on the stage of development reached by the controlling part. The body does not, therefore, retain the same proportions throughout growth, and the relative weights and sizes of given tissues and organs do not remain constant. This differential growth also implies movement of one part relative to another. For example, because of the relatively very small pelvis of the baby, the bladder is an abdominal organ in early childhood; as the pelvis grows, so the bladder sinks down into it.

The third point to notice is that the definitions omit the fact that growth does not cease when maturity is attained. We are all familiar with the continued growth of our skin, nails, and hair, but other less obvious forms of growth also continue throughout adult life. For example, the lining of the alimentary tract is constantly being renewed, and in nearly every tissue and organ there is a recurring cycle of growth, death, and replacement. There may also be processes of disordered growth which result in various forms of tumours in the adult as well as in the child.

Three further points must be made concerning definitions. The first is that the most spectacular phase of growth occurs before birth, and with this we are not directly concerned. The second point relates to the use of the words 'growth' and 'development'. 'Growth' has today assumed the restricted meaning of anatomical and physiological changes, whereas 'development' covers the emergence of psychological attributes, ideas, and understanding, as well as the acquisition of motor and sensory skills. In this sense we shall not discuss 'development', except in a very brief and superficial manner. Thirdly, human growth follows a unique pattern and is very different from that in other mammals and in our near relatives the primates. We will note these points as appropriate but it is beyond the scope of this book to go into too much detail in a very complex area.

Major factors in controlling growth

Clearly, a range of controls must influence the growth of a child. Genetic factors are important, as tall families have tall children and short families tend to have small children. There are also large differences between ethnic groups such as the short Twa (or Pygmy) and the tall Watsui in Africa. Nutrition and environment are also important contributors to the picture, as the child does not grow well if it is starved or denied a good balanced diet or is brought up in poverty. Finally, intrinsic factors such as hormones play a major part in orchestrating the body to grow at the correct rate and appropriate time during childhood and adolescence. What is clear is that the interaction of these different factors can influence the growth and adult size attained by individuals.

Molecular biology, genetics, and growth

Recent developments in genetics and cell and molecular biology have considerably extended our understanding of the function of the cell and its development. The rate of progress in this field is so rapid that any attempt to describe an aspect of growth in detail runs the very real risk of being out of date before pen reaches paper. Hence, this book tries to maintain an approach which describes basic principles and leaves it to readers to develop their own understanding of the latest concepts and developments from other more specialist sources.

Molecular biology investigates the structural, biochemical, and genetic determinates of normal cell function and this clearly will affect our understanding of growth. Evolution repeats successful experiments through each generation, rarely if ever discarding successful developments. Governing this process is natural selection, which has resulted in the conservation of a range of genetic and molecular mechanisms within cells and cell constituents. This has led to control mechanisms for cell division and programmed cell death being similar through a range of species while other processes have developed which are unique to humans. Furthermore, the increasing complexity of the organism as it has evolved has led to the wide range of different systems for regulation of cell functions and existing systems have adapted to new functions. As a result, science has found that mechanisms for cell communication are often very different between species while in other instances the same process can have a totally different outcome if investigated in a wide range of animals. Overlap between these mechanisms is of great biological interest and offers potential opportunities for future developments in the medical sciences in the ongoing battle against disease.

Box 1.1 **Molecular analysis**

It has been the rapid development of molecular laboratory techniques which has led to the recent advances in our understanding of the human genome and the genetic modification of other organisms. Core to this is the isolation and identification of DNA sequences and associated RNA. In essence, this is achieved by applying a number of similar electrophoretic techniques to samples in which the DNA has been cut at specific sites using appropriate enzymes. These are the so-called 'blotting techniques' (Northern blotting, Southern blotting, etc.). The polymerase chain reaction (PCR) is one technique used for cloning the identified sequences DNA which has had a major impact on our understanding of a number of inherited disorders. The full details of these different methods are beyond the scope of this book but it should be appreciated that the techniques have had and will continue to have a major impact on our understanding of how the body functions and grows.

Box 1.2 **The genome project and human genes**

The Human Genome project was established in 1988 as an international collaboration of scientists who would all work together to identify all the sequence of genes that make up the genetic pattern of humans and other animals. Once methods of investigating the nature of DNA had been developed, researchers discovered that DNA naturally has a number of sequence variations that could be easily detected and used as genetic markers. This formed the basis for the systematic programme of mapping and sequencing human genes and by collaboration, resulted in the genome project becoming established. The project will undoubtedly result in our understanding more about the genes that control growth and other physio-logical processes and has contributed to discoveries why some inherited conditions occur, such as cystic fibrosis. Genetic unravelling has also led to opportunities to incorporate human genes into animals such as pigs, raising the possibility of using non-human organs as a source of transplant material—so-called xenotransplantation techniques. Such animal models are called transgenic animals and they provide medical researchers with invalu-able insights into the complex biochemical and physiological processes responsible for abnormal disease conditions as well as growth and growth controlling mechanisms.

Processes of growth

The body consists of cells and intercellular matrix, and both these grow, with the former in size and number, and the latter in amount. When the component cells of a tissue or organ increase in number by dividing, growth is said to be

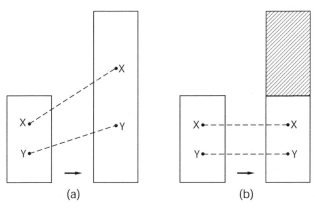

Fig. 1.1 Interstitial (a) and appositional (b) growth. In interstitial growth new material is laid down more or less evenly throughout the block of tissue, so that the distance between the cells X and Y increases as growth takes place. In appositional growth the new material is simply added on top of the old, so that the distance between X and Y remains constant.

multiplicative: when they increase in size, growth is auxetic. When the non-living structural material between the cells is increased in amount, the resultant growth is called accretionary.

A distinction must also be made between interstitial and appositional growth. In the former the tissue grows uniformly throughout its mass, and in the latter the new material is added to the surface of the existing substance (Fig. 1.1).

Cell growth, division, and the cell cycle

It has been estimated that the number of cells in the human adult is of the order of 10^{14}, and all these are ultimately derived from the single fertilized ovum. This may seem a very large number, but only some 45 generations of cell divisions would be sufficient to attain it.

The ovum is a large cell (Fig. 1.3a) and its initial division into two as a result of penetration by the spermatozoon is not preceded by any increase in the amount of cytoplasm it contains. The two daughter cells thus each receive about half the material of the parent cell. After a few generations of division, however, the cells do not divide until they have gone through a phase of apparent inactivity called the interphase. In interphase, cells may grow and enlarge, synthesize cytoplasm and absorb water.

The sequence of growth followed by division is called the cell cycle and is followed by all subsequent generations of cells.

Cell division in the first couple of generations occurs more or less simultaneously in every cell, but after the cells begin growing before dividing, the timing

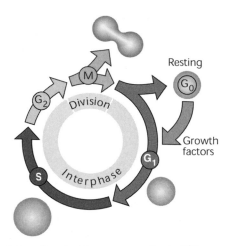

Fig. 1.2 The stages of the cell cycle. M represents mitosis. G^0 is a resting phase and G^1 is the phase through which the cell passes to the stage (S) when DNA synthesis occurs. This is followed by G^2. Growth factors and other signals determine if the cell enters the G^0 or G^1 stages. Growth of the cell occurs throughout G^1 and G^2.

becomes staggered, so that in a given tissue only a small proportion of the cells are engaged in dividing at any one time.

The continuing process of cell division enables the body to grow to adult size by a steady and gradual process and not in fits and starts. Some groups of cells are stimulated to divide while others of apparently equal maturity remain stable, although how this mechanism is controlled is not known.

A cell which is not growing is said to be quiescent, although this term is misleading, for it may be functionally very active.

Most cells in the human body, whether actively dividing or quiescent, are anchored in a fixed position and are surrounded by tissue fluid which supplies them with nutriments. This fluid is derived from the blood. Cells normally do not divide unless they receive a signal to do so. Such a signal arrives in the tissue fluid as a growth factor.

Growth factors are generally proteins or polypeptides produced either locally by certain cells, when they are called paracrine factors, or else by cells in an organ situated at a distance, in which case they are categorized as endocrine factors or hormones (e.g. the growth hormone secreted by the pituitary gland).

The growth factors are captured by receptors situated between the two lipid layers of the plasma membrane surrounding the cell, and following this a signal is transmitted, via one of a number of different chemical mechanisms, depending on the receptor concerned, to genes in the chromosomes of the nucleus. These transmission mechanisms are described under the heading of autocrine growth factors. The growth-controlling genes at which the signal arrives determine the proteins the cell produces, some of which enable it to perform its distinctive functions while others provide it with a protoplasmic skeleton. Growth receptors are proteins, and some are very specific, reacting with only one growth factor; others may accept several, and some require the presence of potentiating substances which do not themselves initiate growth. Cells which respond to a particular growth factor are called its target cells. For example, there is an epidermal growth factor having epithelia as its target, and a macrophage colony-stimulating factor for which the target is the precursor of the monocytes and macrophages of the blood. Other growth factors are trained on multiple targets.

It has been found that cells will not enter the cell cycle and divide unless they are anchored to a surface. The anchorage dependence may well prevent cells displaced from their normal site dividing inappropriately. Other inhibitions to division include the density of the tissue. This is called density-dependent inhibition and suggests that the rate of cell division decreases as the cell population becomes more closely packed. The inhibition can be reversed in culture if cells are placed in an open space. The cause of this inhibition is probably the inadequate supply of local growth factors to the cells and is a major factor in the regulation of growth of the body's tissues, keeping cell populations at an optimal level.

The cell-cycle control system employs a set of growth factor proteins which both initiate and co-ordinate major growth events within the cell during interphase. Consequently, events do not themselves drive the cell cycle but require these proteins in the control system to trigger such an event. Interphase is itself divided into three subphases called G_1, S and G_2 (G refers to gap). Within the G_1 subphase, the cell increases its supply of proteins, increases the number of its internal organelles (including mitochondria and ribosomes) and grows in size. In the S phase, an adequate supply of suitable raw materials is essential to the cell so that deoxyribonucleic acid (DNA) synthesis or replication can take place and the single chromosome present at the start of this phase is reduplicated into a pair of sister chromatids. The duplication of DNA is of the utmost precision, so that when the chromosomes divide at the end of interphase during cell division the chromosomal material passed on to each daughter cell is identical with that contained in the mother cell. The final G_2 phase leads up to actual cell division and is a period of intensive metabolic activity, including the production of proteins essential to the process of cell division.

The checks that occur during the subphases of interphase will block the process unless they are overridden by another stimulating growth signal. While many of these signals are received by the cell control system within the cell, others come as messages from outside the cell, indicating the presence of both a specific molecular signal from other cells and also the appropriate environmental conditions. Most of the inhibition checks occur within the G_1 phase of interphase and require a positive growth factor signal to permit the cell to proceed towards division. If no signal is received, the cell enters a permanent non-dividing state. Such events occur in our muscles and nerve cells in the brain.

Cell division involves two stages. In the first, called mitosis, the nucleus and its contents divide and are equally distributed to the two daughter cells. The second stage, called cytokinesis, involves the division of the cytoplasm of the cell into two by a process called cleavage. Both these stages overlap with one another and are termed the mitotic phase of the cell cycle.

There is a limit to the size a cell can attain, and this limit is set by purely physical and chemical factors. As a spherical cell grows, its volume increases with the cube of the radius, but its surface area only increases with the square of the radius. The volume of the cell determines its biochemical activity, as metabolism goes on throughout its substance, with all the materials necessary for this activity passing through the surface membrane. Therefore, as the cell grows, its biochemical function becomes more and more restricted through a relative lack of raw materials and energy, and eventually some resulting chemical stimulus causes it to divide. What this stimulus might be is unknown: cell size is not the only factor, as amoebae can be induced to divide when they are well below the weight at which division normally occurs. However, an amoeba less than one-third of this weight will not divide whatever encouragement it is given. The stimulus to division originates in the cytoplasm rather than in the nucleus, and in multi-nucleated cells all the nuclei divide synchronously.

The restriction on size of individual cells can to some extent be overcome if the cell alters its spherical shape by elongating (nerve cells), flattening (epithelial cells), or folding up its surface membrane (intestinal cells), for in all these ways surface area can be increased without much change in volume. Cells in closely packed tissues do not have much option, since the laws of physics cause them to tend to take up a shape which partitions the space available with a maximum economy of surface area. Lord Kelvin showed that an assembly of regular 14-sided figures (tetrakaidekahedra) fits these conditions best, and this is the form which is seen in the interior of a mass of soap bubbles. A similar arrangement of rather more irregular sided figures is found in animal tissues (Fig. 1.4).

Another factor which may play a part in determining the time at which a cell must divide is the ratio between the size of the cell as a whole and the size of its nucleus. The nucleus consists mostly of chromatin, and does not increase in size at the same rate as the cytoplasm. The surface area of the nucleus, through which all interchange between the nucleus and the cytoplasm must take place, thus becomes inadequate to allow proper control of the cytoplasm by the nucleus, and it has been suggested that cells divide in an attempt to keep a fairly constant ratio between the amounts of the material in the nucleus

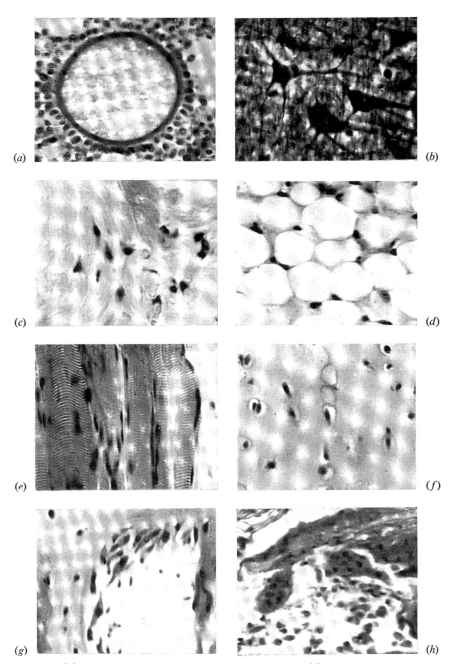

Fig. 1.3 (a) a secondary oocyte; (b) multipolar nerve cells; (c) fibroblasts from a healing wound; (d) fat cells; (e) muscle fibres; (f) cartilage cells; (g) osteoblasts within bone; (h) multinucleated osteoclasts.

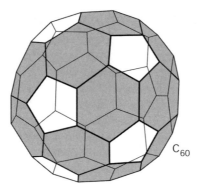

C_{60}

Fig. 1.4 A five-sided structure fits well together. This is an example used by the 'Bukeyball' of Carbon 60. Living cells adopt more irregular shapes so as to fit closely together.

and in the cytoplasm. Just as a cell can partly escape from the limitations to its growth by altering its shape, so the nucleus can allow some further increase in cytoplasm by becoming flattened or lobulated, although again there is a limit to the scope which such manoeuvres allow.

The processes of growth and cell division are complementary and inter-dependent. Growth of a cell beyond a certain size is impossible, and further growth of the tissue of which the cell is a part involves a temporary reduction of the size of its cells by the process of division.

In the same way, a period of growth must precede cell division, otherwise the size of the cells would be progressively reduced.

During the maturation of the male and female sex cells, the diploid number of chromosomes in the nucleus ($2n$) is reduced to the haploid number (n) because, in the process of meiosis, the chromosomes segregate into two groups, one of which passes into each daughter cell; the chromosomes do not divide. (In humans, $n = 23$.)

At fertilization, the diploid number is restored (Fig. 1.5) and the offspring of the fertilized ovum maintain the diploid number because, as already mentioned, each chromosome splits during mitosis longitudinally into two halves, one of which passes into each daughter cell.

Occasionally, however, somatic cells with $3n$, $4n$, $5n$, etc., chromosomes are found, and such cells are said to be polyploid. Although such cells are not common in the human body, they can occur, particularly in the liver.

Even-numbered polyploidy (e.g. $4n$, $8n$) can be produced by the chromosomes dividing preparatory to a mitosis which does not take place. Odd-numbered polyploidy, which is much rarer, may be due to anomalies in the nuclear spindle at the time of mitosis. Polyploid cells can accommodate an amount of cytoplasm which is more or less proportional to the amount of nuclear material.

The DNA produced during the S subphase of interphase can be 'labelled'

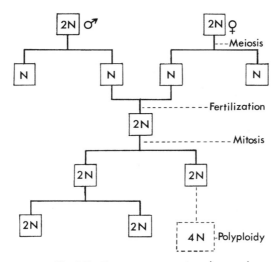

Fig. 1.5 Chromosome numbers (see text).

with tritiated thymidine, and autoradiography can then give an estimate of the rate of cell proliferation in different tissues. This is possible because the amount of DNA per cell is constant, and an increase in the DNA content of a tissue or organ therefore indicates an increase in the number of cells it contains. But it is known that cells can accumulate DNA at a very much slower rate than that found in tissues where active cell division is taking place, and there may be a slow turnover of DNA content quite apart from cell division.

A simpler method depends on the fact that the process of mitosis is readily identifiable histologically (Fig. 1.6a). The number of dividing cells per thousand cells of a given tissue is known as its mitotic index, and this index (and thus the rate of growth) is influenced by many factors, such as age, sex, weight, diet, temperature, and time of day.

Cell differentiation

Not only do cells divide and grow, they also tend to become 'differentiated'. In the very early stages of pregnancy, before the pre-embryo develops from the cells of the fertilized ovum, dissection out of individual daughter or grand-daughter cells has shown that these cells can prove capable of giving rise to a whole normal animal. Such cells are referred to as 'multipotent'. Later, dividing cells in the developing pre-embryo rapidly lose this capacity and become 'committed' to a certain specialized line of development by beginning to synthesize different proteins. As the embryo develops further, the majority of committed cells become further differentiated, so that their offspring ultimately give rise to specific tissues such as muscle, bone, etc.

Every cell is endowed with the same complement of genes, which are transmitted at the time of cell division from the mother to the daughter cells, and which determine cell function by dictating the synthesis of specific proteins. It therefore follows that in a differentiated cell some of the genes must have been prevented from exerting their effects ('selective repression'), and others must have had their effects unblocked ('selective activation'). Further, the changes must be stable, so that the progeny of a differentiated cell inherit the new pattern; under normal circumstances a given type of differentiated cell 'breeds true'. Nevertheless, under special conditions, cells can give rise to products quite foreign to their normal role; for example, fully differentiated liver cells, which normally produce albumin, may in diseased states or in culture give rise to collagen. Additionally, there is evidence that the maternal environment may influence cell development in the embryo by the process of imprinting in which genes are switched on or off as required. Evidence supporting this concept has come from work in mice where mouse embryos which were transferred to genetically different mothers tend to be born resembling the surrogate mother. The implications for humans is not known at present, although there is a suggestion that surrogate mothers can pass on defects to the fetus they are carrying.

The factors which lead to a cell becoming differentiated are still unclear, but they appear to include the effect that other cells in the body can have in which there is evidence of 'messenger proteins' exerting an influence at a distance on cells. This mechanism is supported by experiments in which embryonic cells removed from an experimental animal are cultured in appropriate media and continue to grow and multiply without differentiating further. Similar cells left in their original site continue to multiply and become differentiated.

Other influences on the differentiation of a cell can include its responses to growth-producing stimuli. For example, the sex hormones secreted at the time of puberty have a much greater effect on the growth of certain tissues than on others, and the secondary sexual characteristics are produced by this selective stimulation.

The tools by which science might recognize that differentiation has taken place are still relatively crude, often having to rely largely on visual appearances under the light or electron microscope. When the fully differentiated cell has the task of elaborating an easily recognizable product, such as pigment, it is simple to detect the final stages. But the precursors of such a cell may contain little structural evidence relating to the activities of their descendants, and attempts to detect the specialized apparatus with which it is assumed they are equipped eventually peter out in failure as one traces the ancestral line back towards the ovum.

The first stages of differentiation are probably chemical in nature, but very little indeed has been discovered about them, although sometimes chemical changes can be detected before structural changes become apparent, for example, in the developing heart of the chick.

Undifferentiated cells tend to be nondescript in appearance, to be arranged in random patterns, to have relatively simple structure and functions, and to be highly adaptable under differing environmental conditions. In contrast, differentiated cells tend to be regular in appearance, to have a complex structure and specialized functions, and to be much more rigid and unadaptable. Some examples of differentiated cells are shown in Fig. 1.3, and their appearances are often strikingly dissimilar. Nevertheless, the one true criterion of differentiation is function; a cell which retains only a single functional potentiality must be regarded as fully differentiated whatever its appearance.

Differentiation and multiplication tend to be mutually exclusive, and the more specialized a cell is, the less likely it is to be able to divide. An extreme example is the erythrocyte, which, in the course of specialization to a respiratory function, loses its nucleus, and with it any hope of division or indeed of repairing any damage it may suffer.

As cells differentiate they begin to carry out their specific chemical operations, and the results of their activity may contribute to the processes of growth. For example, the cells of the thyroid gland produce secretion which accumulates locally in the gland, causing it to enlarge by passive distension, and at the same time circulates throughout the body via the bloodstream with profound results on the growth of many tissues and organs.

Regulation of cell populations

Tissues may be roughly classified into those in which there is a very active turnover of the cell population, those with a moderate turnover, and those with none. To the first group belong those tissues in which cells are constantly being lost or destroyed, and in which the total mass is kept constant; it includes epidermis and its derivatives, the lining of the gut, endometrium, transitional epithelium, the blood-forming tissues, and the cells producing the male and female sex cells. In such tissues the new cells are derived from special, relatively undifferentiated 'stem' cells which are collectively known as the growth fraction of the tissue.

These more primitive cells retain the ability to reproduce themselves without becoming differentiated; there is thus a constant pool of stem cells available, and in this way the differentiated population can be maintained at a steady level. Precise control of the system is vital, for the multiplication of undifferentiated stem cells must be exactly balanced by the input of differentiated cells.

An example of a control mechanism of this kind is the ability of the body to maintain the approximately constant number of erythrocytes in the bloodstream despite the immense daily destruction (estimated at about 350 000 million) of these cells. Like the other types of blood corpuscles, the erythrocytes are ultimately derived from multipotent stem cells in the bone marrow, which give rise to the secondary progenitor stem cells of different lineages—erythrocytes, lymphocytes, platelets, etc. A large family of different growth factors stimulate differentiation in the various directions required. For example, the glycoprotein erythropoietin, which is mainly made in the kidney, arouses the multiplication of the stem cells of the erythrocyte line and their differentiation into erythrocyte precursors. It is thus a major factor in erythrocyte production, and biosynthetic erythropoietin has recently been produced for clinical use in cases of anaemia arising from kidney failure.

If the oxygen tension in the blood is reduced, as when someone goes to live at a high altitude, the stem cells in the marrow are stimulated to produce more erythrocytes, the number being adjusted precisely to the respiratory needs. A similar increase in stem cell division in the marrow follows loss of blood by haemorrhage. We can say that the system of growth factors responds to lack of oxygen or to some chemical stimulus resulting from lack of oxygen, but this merely serves to clothe our ignorance in words; we have no idea of the basic processes involved or of the antagonistic controls which prevent the system from manufacturing so many erythrocytes that the viscosity of the blood would rise dangerously.

In the second group there is no necessary loss of cells as a result of function, and the cell population thus does not constantly require to be restored. Growth in such organs as the liver, the kidney, and the exocrine and endocrine glands occurs by division of the functioning cells themselves, and turnover is relatively slow. Nevertheless, their apparently specialized cells can, if appropriately stimulated, become temporarily able to divide and reproduce at a remarkable rate, and this is particularly important in the repair of injuries (Chapter 9).

The third group is small but important. Somatic muscle and nervous tissue grow by cell division only in the early stages of their development; further growth is produced merely by enlargement of the existing cells, which can—at least theoretically—live as long as the body lives. This inhibition of division is due to the presence of growth inhibitors, particularly in the brain, which stop cells dividing.

Growth of intercellular matrix

In the early embryo the intercellular matrix is scanty and amorphous. Later it increases in quantity, and comes to contain viscous substances which give it a gel-like consistency and enable it to hold a large amount of fluid. Chief among these substances are hyaluronic acid, a polysaccharide which retains water tenaciously and tends to become more viscous the more calcium is present in the fluid, and chondroitin sulphate, which is a firmer gel than hyaluronic acid and is particularly plentiful in cartilage.

Later still, as connective tissue cells become differentiated, the matrix harbours fibres of two types. The more numerous of these are composed of collagen, a scleroprotein which by its ubiquity accounts for about one-third of all the protein in the body. Collagen fibres are laid down where firmness is needed—for example, in bone, skin, and tendon—and occur in bundles about 1–100 μm in diameter. Individual fibres do not branch, but connections exist between bundles because fibres often leave one bundle and join another: they take a straight or slightly wavy course through the matrix (Fig. 1.6b).

Collagen fibres are closely associated with fibroblasts, which synthesize a predecessor protein called tropocollagen. This is extruded from the cell, and the microfibrils which go to form collagen are then assembled in the extracellular spaces. However, collagen fibres appear in the matrix of the embryo at a time when very few cells, let alone fibroblasts, are present. Sulphated polysaccharides may play an essential part in their formation, and other factors are known to be involved: for instance, vitamin C deficiency leads to defective collagen formation.

The second type of fibre is the elastic fibre, about which less is known. It is generally agreed that it is produced extracellularly, and the presence of collagen in the neighbourhood may be necessary for its formation. In the majority of situations the parent cell is probably the fibroblast, but in the walls of elastic arteries it is believed that smooth muscle may be responsible. Elastic fibres are thinner than collagen fibres (0.2–1 μm in diameter), and branch freely; the individual fibres are relatively straight (Fig. 1.6b). They have a core of the protein elastin, surrounded by microfibrils which show beading. The first indication of the advent of an elastic fibre is the deposition of parallel arrays of microfibrils in the matrix: the core of the fibre is a later addition.

The formation of matrix and fibres continues throughout the whole period of growth, and is a vital factor in the repair of injuries (Chapter 9). As growth proceeds, the matrix loses some of its water content, and important changes occur in it as old age advances (Chapter 11).

Phases of growth

There are four main phases in the growth of the body. In the early embryo, everything is subordinated to growth, and there is little differentiation of function. This phase merges into a second one during which a balance is struck between growth and differentiated functional activity. This phase continues throughout childhood and ceases at maturity with the attainment of adulthood. During adulthood, a third phase supervenes, in which the goal is functional activity, and growth becomes a matter of making good losses occurring through wear and tear. The last phase occurs in old age, when growth becomes insufficient to maintain equilibrium, so that cells are lost without replacement, and functions may become inefficient as a result (Chapter 11). Finally, growth ceases with the death of the component tissues. In every phase the balance between growth and function can be upset by the advent of injury, which stimulates the growth necessary to effect repairs.

Before birth, cell division is the main cause of growth, although other processes occur also. After birth multiplicative growth continues, but the importance of auxetic and accretionary growth increases. The extreme example of the contrast between antenatal and postnatal growth is afforded by the nervous system, in which it is thought that no new nerve cells appear after the sixth month of fetal life. If this is so, we already have at birth all the nerve cells we can ever possess. In the postnatal phase of growth the nerve cells add to the amount of cytoplasm surrounding their nuclei, and use some of this additional material to extend their peripheral processes and increase the number and intricacy of their communications with other nerve cells.

The logistics of cell division during the four phases of growth are naturally complicated, for different proportions of stem cells and differentiated cells must be produced at different stages. If every stem cell divided into two more stem cells, as in the earliest stages of embryonic development, the embryo would become a mass of unspecialized cells. If, on the other hand, every stem cell divided into two differentiated cells incapable of further division, growth would abruptly come to a halt. The controls and checks which orderly growth requires can be illustrated by a specific example.

In the adult phase of growth of the skin, cells which are lost from the surface by attrition are replaced by the activity of stem cells in the germinative layer in the depths of the epidermis (see Fig. 9.1, p. 172).

Neglecting programmed cell death, these cells must produce 50% of offspring which are differentiated and gradually proceed to the surface to be shed, and 50% of offspring which remain as stem cells to continue the process of growth replacement. Any other proportion would mean that the skin would either show signs of overgrowth, or else fail to replace wear and tear and so become thinner. Of course this does not imply that every individual stem cell in the germinative layer must divide into one stem cell and one differentiated cell; all it means is that the overall result of cell division must be equal numbers of stem and differentiated cells.

What seems to happen in practice is that the growth fraction produces many more cells than are needed for maintenance, and that the superfluous cells then undergo programmed destruction.

This is the situation in the adult phase of growth, but in the first two phases the number of stem cells in the germinative layer must increase, so that the growth of the skin keeps pace with that of the body which it covers. At the same time the skin grows in thickness, so that more differentiated cells must also be produced by the activity of yet more stem cells. Further, the skin has to become thicker in some places than in others, so that local as well as general controls are necessary. In contrast, the thickness of the skin diminishes in old age because the stem cells are unable any longer to keep pace with the surface losses. In all these phases the fine adjustment maintaining the balance between division and differentiation is a razor edge between 'normal' and 'abnormal'. If the adjustment becomes disorganized, uncontrolled local or general growth may take over, or further growth may cease (Chapter 10).

There is some rather circumstantial evidence that suggests the existence of a negative-feedback mechanism which inhibits growth and cell division in the germinative basal layers of the skin. These substances, if they exist, are called chalones and they work by binding to adrenaline and inhibiting mitosis in the cell. This effect maintains the balance between cell division and differentiation.

There is every likelihood that growth and replacement in other tissues and organs, such as the wall of the gut, the kidneys, and the lungs, depend on similar negative-feedback mechanisms. It has not yet been conclusively proved that each of these systems is specific for its own particular tissue, but this is probably the case. On this view, the hormonal control of cycles of growth and death such as the menstrual cycle is only a more generalized extension of the universal local chemical control systems which keep mitosis and function in balance.

Enough has perhaps been said to indicate that cell division is subject to controls at each stage of development, that some of these controls are highly specialized, and that many of them still remain to be explained and understood.

Growth curves

The amount of growth achieved depends on the time for which growth proceeds and on the speed of growth per unit time.

Among the primates, the duration of postnatal growth seems to be correlated with the age at which sexual maturity is reached; the greater this age, the longer the period of growth. Growth in lemurs lasts for 2 or 3 years, in monkeys for 7 or 8 years, in great apes for 10 or 11 years, and in humans for up to 20 or more years.

Measurements taken on a single individual at intervals can be plotted against time to produce a graph of progress (Fig. 1.7), whether they are derived from the whole body or from one of its component parts. A graph of this sort is sometimes called a 'distance curve', as any point on it indicates the distance travelled along the road to maturity. The curve flattens out to a plateau as growth ceases.

Another way of presenting the same data is shown in Fig. 1.8, in which the increments of growth (the amounts added in specific time intervals) are plotted

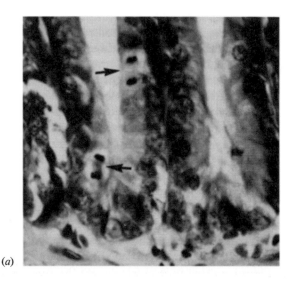

(a)

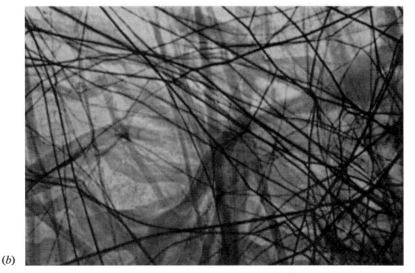

(b)

Fig. 1.6 (a) Mitotic figures. Two mitotic figures (arrowed) in the wall of the intestine. (Original photomicrograph by kind permission of Dr. N. Thomas.)
(b) Collagen and elastic fibres. A spread of mesentery showing collagen fibres (thick, pale bundles which do not branch) and elastic fibres (thin, branching, darkly stained). (Original photomicrograph by kind permission of Dr. N. Thomas.)

against time. Such a curve shows the variation in the rate of growth with time, and is therefore known as a 'velocity curve'. The curve tends to zero as growth ceases.

If a growth curve is derived from a single individual, or from repeated measurements on the same group of individuals, it is said to be based on 'longitudinal' data. Such information is naturally difficult to get, as every

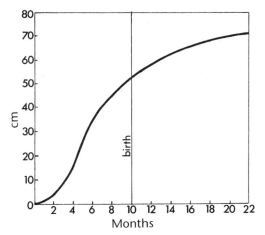

Fig. 1.7 Distance curve for stature before and after birth. Each point on the graph represents the mean height of several embryos or children of that particular age: the curve is therefore said to be derived from cross-sectional data (see text). (From Thompson, D'Arcy W. (1942). *Growth and form* (2nd edn). Cambridge University Press, London, by kind permission of the publishers.)

subject must report at regular intervals to be measured, and in consequence gaps in the records are only too common. It also requires a great deal of patience, as results cannot be evaluated for several years. It is much easier to obtain what are called 'horizontal' or 'cross-sectional' data. Measurements are made of several children in each age group, and these are then combined to form a cross-sectional picture of the various age-groups in the community at the time of the investigation. In such work, the sample can be controlled accurately; as each child is measured only once there is no difficulty about children not returning to be measured, and the results are immediately available. Nevertheless, they are not so useful from a statistical point of view as are longitudinal data, and may actually be misleading if one wishes to investigate such matters as changes in development or alterations in velocity (Fig. 2.6, p. 31). For such work, longitudinal studies are essential.

'Mixed longitudinal' investigations are longitudinal ones in which some of the children dropped out and had to be replaced by others. Instead of having to discard all information obtained from those who did not complete the whole course, the investigator can use special statistical methods to obtain a meaningful result.

Mathematical models of growth

The growth curve, such as that shown in Fig. 1.7, presents an obvious challenge to the mathematically minded and consequently, over the years, many attempts have been made to express growth curves in mathematical form. As a consequence, while over 200 mathematical models have been devised to represent certain aspects of growth and development, about six are widely used to analyse growth patterns. A very brief discussion of some of these is given here as an indication of the range of solutions to the problem involved.

The initial stages of growth after fertilization involve cell division only, and proceed in geometrical progression, one cell giving rise to two, two to four, four to eight, and so on. We have already noted that growth gradually slows down towards a halt as maturity is approached, and it follows that the curve of growth from the ovum to the adult must be S-shaped. The part of it which describes growth after birth results, in varying combinations, from cell division, cell enlargement, and the production of matrix. The first of these factors suggests geometrical progression and the other two suggest arithmetical progression: it will already be clear that no simple equation is likely to help us very much.

If cells are grown in tissue culture, the initial geometrical progression does not continue indefinitely, for the supply of foodstuffs is not unlimited, and the environment is progressively polluted by the waste products of the cells. There is thus a gradual slowing down of multiplication, until finally it stops. If there is no renewal of the environment, the cells resulting from the process of multiplication must eventually die, so that their number gradually returns to zero. If, however, the environment is continuously renewed, the population of cells ultimately approaches the maximum which the available volume or medium will support, so producing an S-shaped curve known as the curve of logistic growth (Fig. 1.9), which is described by the equation:

$$W = \frac{a}{1 + be^{-kt}}$$

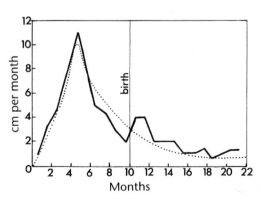

Fig. 1.8 Velocity curve for stature before and after birth: derived from the same data as Fig. 1.7. Each point on the graph represents the mean increase in length during that particular month. (From Thompson, D'Arcy W. (1942). *Growth and form* (2nd edn). Cambridge University Press, London, by kind permission of the publishers.)

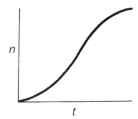

Fig. 1.9 Curve of logistic growth. n = number of cells present; t = time.

where W is weight and t is time, and a, b, and k are constants. This type of curve can be adapted to fit human growth data and expresses the idea that the rate of growth is dependent on the number of cells present and on the concentration of the available food supply.

Early attempts to modify development curves of this type allowed Count in 1943 to produce three models which fitted data between 0 and 7 years, 7 and 13 years, and ages over 13. This produced results which were in close accordance with biological growth. By following endocrine events during growth, later work introduced four phase models which obtained a fairly good fit of events within the growth cycle, both prepubertally and postpubertally.

These models employed a type of S-shaped curve called the Gompertz curve, originally devised in 1825 for use in actuarial tables. A simple form may be written:

$$W = ae^{-be^{-kt}}$$

and expresses the idea that an organism loses, in equal small intervals of time, equal proportions of its remaining power to grow.

Figure 1.10a shows the distance curve and Fig. 1.10b the velocity curve derived from the Gompertz equation written above; they may be compared with Figs 1.7 and 1.8. The acceleration curve derived from this equation (Fig. 1.10c) has a positive, followed by a negative phase, returning to zero with the cessation of growth.

In experimental work it is sometimes mathematically convenient to plot the logarithm of the measurement against time, thereby producing what is known as a 'specific growth' curve. This is a record of how the tissue is multiplying itself; if it does so at a constant rate, the curve becomes a straight line. Figure 1.10d shows the specific growth curve of the Gompertz equation, and Figs 1.10e and 1.10f the velocity and acceleration curves derived from it. If the multiplication rate were constant, the velocity curve would be a constant, and the acceleration would become zero.

Other equations with less readily understandable implications than the Gompertz or logistic curves have also been fitted to human growth data. For example, it is found experimentally that growth from about the age of 1 year to about the age of 10 years can be fitted fairly well by a curve of the form:

$$W = a + bt + c \log t,$$

although the biological meaning of the terms is far from clear. However, the real problem remains with transition periods between one growth period to another as it was recognized that the use of time within the equation was misleading; children's growth patterns actually follow a time-independent biological timetable.

This can be overcome by using more complex logistic curves, such as the curve devised by Bock in 1973 which used the summation of two logistic curves. One curve describes the adolescent growth spurt while the other adds in the component attributed to prepubertal growth. Addition of a third component effectively divides the prepubertal period into two parts allowing us an accurate means to describe infantile, juvenile, and adolescent growth precisely.

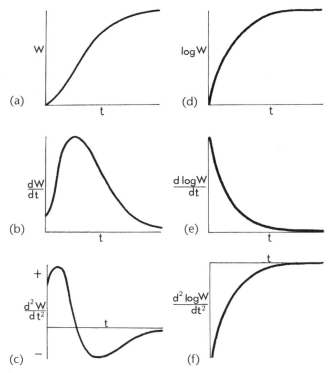

Fig. 1.10 A Gompertz function (a) Distance curve; (b) velocity curve; (c) acceleration curve; (d) curve of specific growth; (e) velocity curve of specific growth; (f) acceleration curve of specific growth. The scales of the ordinates have been adjusted to make the height of all the graphs the same. W=weight; t=time. [From Medawar, P.B. (1945). Size, shape and age. In Essays on growth and form. Clarendon Press, Oxford, by kind permission of the author and publishers.)

Refinement of mathematical modelling by Preece and Bains in 1978 produced a new curve which is based on the assumption that the rate of growth of the individual is not one of proportionality but is a function of age. This now allows elements relating to differential growth to be included in the mathematical model. The result is a model which relates more closely to reality by allowing for children that grow at different speeds, either relatively slowly or relatively quickly. The Preece–Bains model also is valuable as it allows calculation of events such as the minimum prepubertal velocity with reasonable accuracy. It has found widespread application in research which compares populations with one another.

No model is perfect as arbitrary events in growth are force-fitted into the shape of the model. Events such as the juvenile growth spurt may be overlooked or missed and this may be important if the child has a growth problem.

As mathematics and computer programs have developed, more and more complex equations have been devised which try to mimic growth more closely. This is a highly specialized area, is often difficult for the non-mathematician to follow, and clearly beyond the remit of this book to consider in detail. The newer models allow functions such as neuroendocrine development to be analysed and are routinely applied to describe growth curves in general and the adolescent spurt in particular. Many of these equations are available within statistical packages for use on computers. By consultation of specialist publications by Goldstein, Tanner, and others, the reader can gain more insight into an area of great interest to researchers into growth.

2 Growth in height and weight

With sobs and tears he sorted out
Those of the largest size
Lewis Carroll

Growth in height

Growth curves and growth charts

The human ovum measures about l00 μm in diameter, and is just visible to the naked eye. At birth, a baby is about 50 cm (20 in) long—roughly 5000 times as long as the ovum. Further growth in height after birth may take the adult to a height of (say) 175 cm (5 ft 9 in)—three and a half times the length of the baby.

The process of growth is not uniform in human throughout life. Each region and part of the body can be shown to have its own growth rate and this can vary according to age as well. For height, the maximum rate of increase actually occurs in the fetus. It reaches a maximum of approximately 1.5 mm a day at 4 months after fertilization and then progressively slows down for the rest of the period of pregnancy. However, at birth this rate of growth is still rapid if compared with older children but a decrease in height gain in fact continues until the child reaches about 4 years of age.

One of the earliest growth records was that of Gueneau de Montbeillard. Count Philibert de Montbeillard measured the height of his son Gueneau from his birth on 11th April 1759 until 30th January 1777, a period of almost 18 years, at approximately semi-annual intervals and obtained data which represented the first recorded example of growth in a child throughout the growing period. The results were then published by Georges de Buffon in his book *Historie Naturelle* in 1777 (see Fig. 2.1).

Buffon also observed that growth occurred more in the summer and that there was a clear diurnal variation in height. These comments show that Buffon was the discoverer of the seasonal differences in growth in humans.

The figures were later republished in 1927 by Scammon as 'The first Seriatim study of human growth' in the *American Journal of Physical Anthropology*.

It is also well known that the season of the year can influence the rate of growth in many children, being faster in spring and summer than in autumn

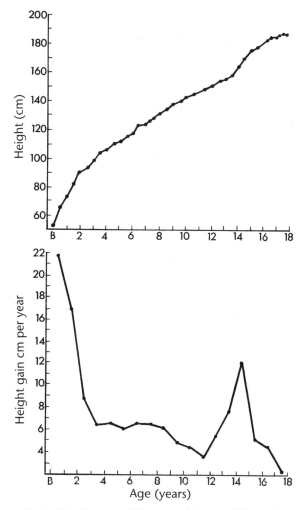

Fig. 2.1 Growth in height. Progress of the son of Count Philibert de Montbeillard from birth to the age of 18 years. Upper graph, distance curve showing height reached at each age: lower graph, velocity curve, showing annual increments in height. (From Tanner, J. M. (1962). *Growth at adolescence* (2nd edn). Blackwell Scientific Publications Ltd., Oxford, by kind permission of the author and publishers.)

and winter, although this rate change can be small and is often only clearly revealed in children during puberty.

There are several problems and difficulties which can affect the measurement of height. In the baby and young child, it is desirable to use supine length or reclining length rather than standing height for the practical reason that standing is either impossible or difficult to maintain at these ages. Special measuring equipment has been developed for the purpose. For older children and all adults, standing height is the accepted measurement generally used (see box 2.1 for technique). The most accurate and valid results can only be obtained when the equipment used is rigid and cannot move.

Height depends to a considerable extent on both the natural curvatures in the vertebral column as well as the width of the intervertebral discs. The discs become compressed by the gravitational strain imposed by the weight of the upper part of the body as soon as an individual gets up in the morning and this continues as the day goes on, with the result that, unless the subject spends the day in bed, he measures less in the evening than he does in the morning. Disc compression has been shown to drive out fluid from the disc structure, reducing its height; the fluid returns when the subject retires to bed and lies down, removing the effect of gravity. This diurnal variation has been shown to be as much as 2 cm, even in children. Thus, it is essential that all measurements of height should be made at the same time of day if at all possible.

Height is also affected by the forces acting on the spine from muscles which maintain normal posture and upright stance. Any condition, such as the early stages of muscular dystrophy, which may weaken this force can alter the overall height. Also, abnormal spinal curvatures such as scoliosis and the curvature secondary to osteoporosis can affect the individual's height.

Finally, it is most desirable that the same person should make every measurement, so that systematic errors of technique or interpretation may be minimized. This is not always easy or even practical when dealing with large numbers. Equally important is the need for the measurer to ensure the accuracy of their technique by the collection of data on the reproducibility of measurements. This particular aspect of growth measurement is often over-looked but will often illustrate how much more satisfactory it is for a single individual to undertake the measurements.

Under the best circumstances the error in measuring an individual is anything up to 3 mm.

Box 2.1 **Measurement of height**

To obtain the most accurate measurement of height which reduce any errors to the minimum, a standard anthropometric method should be adopted. The subject should stand on a firm horizontal floor with their heels against a solid vertical wall and be measured with the aid of a flat horizontal surface rather than a thin bar. A standard posture for the subject must be employed, with the lower border of the orbits level with the external auditory meati of the ears. This is called the Frankfort plane. The examiner should press upwards on the mastoid processes and tell the subject to make him or herself as tall as possible. In children, it is important to ensure they do not rise up on their toes when the pressure is applied.

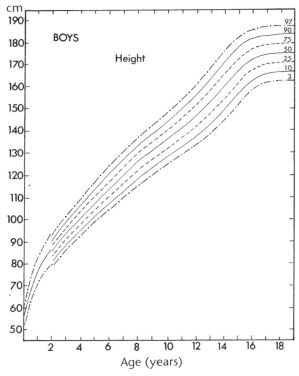

Fig. 2.2 Cross-sectional standards for height attained at each age (English boys). The central line represents the mean, or 50th centile. The two dashed lines above and below it represent the 75th and 25th centiles respectively—i.e. 25 per cent of the sample fell below the lower line and 25 per cent above the upper line. Other centile lines are also provided. (Modified from Tanner, J. M., Whitehouse, R. H., and Takaishi, M. (1966). *Archives of Disease in Childhood*, **41**, 454–71, by kind permission of the authors and the editor.)

Growth charts

Given adequate data from a sufficiently large group of children, usually at least 1000, it is possible to construct a chart which shows the relationship of height to age in the group studied (Figs 2.2 and 2.3). However, there is a considerable spread in the figures for a given age due to the individual variation of the subjects in the sample. This range can be highlighted by the introduction of centile lines on to the chart which employ statistics to indicate the percentages of children whose heights lay on or below the labelled line. Thus, 25% of the group had heights which lay on or below the 25th centile line. Such charts are of course cross-sectional, and it must be stressed that the centile lines do not correspond with, or even lie parallel to, the distance growth curve of any particular child. Longitudinal measurements on an individual (Fig. 2.4) yield growth curves of substantially different shape, and the

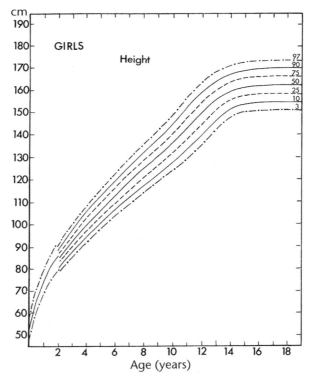

Fig. 2.3 Cross-sectional standards for height attained at each age (English girls). Centiles as in Fig. 2.2. (Modified from Tanner, J. M., Whitehouse, R. H., and Takaishi, M. (1966). *Archives of Disease in Childhood*, **41**, 454–71, by kind permission of the authors and the editor.)

plots for healthy children often cross centile lines, particularly in the first 2 years of life.

Charts of height for age are invaluable in paediatrics, but their use requires a good deal of caution. If a measurement shows that a child lies below the 3% centile—i.e. that he/she is smaller than 97% of the children in the 'standard' group—there is a temptation to suppose that his/her progress has been 'abnormal', and that there must be something wrong with him/her. In the first place we must be sure that we are comparing like with like, for children in different circumstances do not necessarily grow in the same way, and a chart derived from American children may look very different from a chart representing the growth of Indian children.

Growth charts require regular updating, for the children of today may be considerably taller at a given age than the children of 20 years ago. The charts used in this book are derived from the original standard work of Tanner, Whitehouse and Takaishi and these standards have had to be updated by data

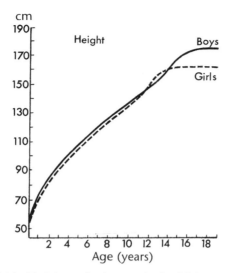

Fig. 2.4 Typical individual height-attained curves for English boys and girls. From Tanner, J. M., Whitehouse, R. H., and Takaishi, M. (1966). *Archives of Disease in Childhood*, **41**, 454–71, by kind permission of the authors and the editor.)

collected from more recent studies. Growth surveys undertaken in Edinburgh found children were considerably taller than the Tanner standards and work carried out in Liverpool has demonstrated considerable average height differences between inner city children and children from more affluent suburbs. Work in Leeds has looked at the growth rates of children from ethnic minorities.

However, it is important to note that even when the appropriate chart is used, we can only say that a child outside the 3% line is 'unusual'—after all, one child in every 33 of the 'standard' group also fell outside this parameter. The evidence of the standard chart is only one piece among many: for example, the family history is equally important, for there are many genetic deviations among growth patterns and these can include conditions such as familial short stature.

It is generally accepted by growth investigators that the best way to record height and other growth parameter measurements is by using standard deviation scores (SDS). The SDS is calculated by subtracting the mean height of the group from the measured height and then dividing the result by the standard deviation of the group mean. A value of zero indicates that the individual is exactly the same height as the mean, and a positive or a negative value shows the degree of tallness or shortness relative to the mean.

Variations in growth rates with age

In the first year after birth, body length increases by about 50 per cent to

75 cm (about 30 in), and in the second year another 12–13 cm (about 5 in) or so are added. Thereafter, growth in height settles down to a rate of about 5–6 cm every year. However, this growth is not at a regular rate as it is known to be episodic during infancy, where increases in length by 0.5–2.5 cm in a few days can be followed by quite long periods where no growth seems occurs at all. The causes of this episodic growth are not known. It is also worth noting that periods of illness can also slow down growth to unmeasurable rates; after recovery from the illness, the child exhibits a period of catch-up growth during which the growth rate can be as much as 400 times greater than normal. Once the previous growth curve is achieved, the accelerated growth rate slows to normal. Again, the mechanisms behind these changes are not understood.

The 'absolute' growth rate is defined as the amount of growth in a given period divided by the length of the period. The 'relative' rate is obtained by dividing the absolute rate by the initial height and expressing the result as a percentage. Thus, a child 120 cm tall who grew 9 cm in a year and a half would have an absolute growth rate of 6 cm/year, and a relative rate of 5% year.

As the individual child enters the period around puberty, the fairly steady rate of increase in height rises suddenly and markedly. This is termed the adolescent spurt. Unfortunately, this spurt in height is not easily discernible in cross-sectional distance curves of growth, but becomes much more evident in individual longitudinal curves (Fig. 2.4), and is shown very strikingly in longitudinal velocity curves (Fig. 2.5).

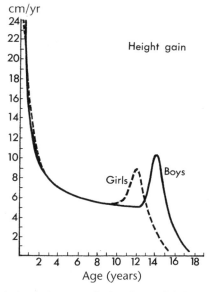

Fig. 2.5 Typical individual velocity curves for height: English boys and girls. (From Tanner, J. M., Whitehouse, R. H., and Takaishi, M. (1966). *Archives of Disease in Childhood*, **41**, 454–71, by kind permission of the authors and the editor.)

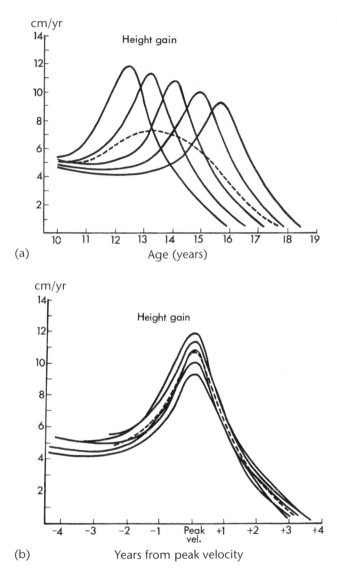

(a)

(b)

Fig. 2.6 Adolescent spurts in height. (A) Individual velocity curves of five boys. The dashed curve is obtained by averaging the individual values at each age. Notice how this average curve fails to show the dramatic nature of the spurt in the individual case. (B) The same curves superimposed so that their peak velocities coincide (see text). (From Tanner, J. M., Whitehouse, R. H., and Takaishi, M. (1966). *Archives of Disease in Childhood*, **41**, 454–71, by kind permission of the authors and the editor.)

The adolescent growth spurt normally begins about the age of $10\frac{1}{2}$–11 years in girls and $12\frac{1}{2}$–13 years in boys, although wide variations are possible (Fig. 2.6); for example, the timing of the onset of the male spurt ranges from $10\frac{1}{2}$ years to 16 years. In both sexes it lasts for 2–$2\frac{1}{2}$ years. During the spurt, boys

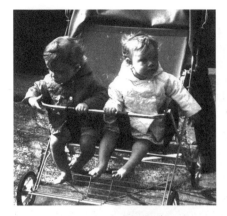
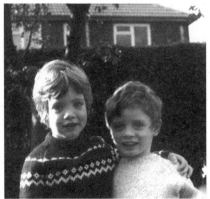
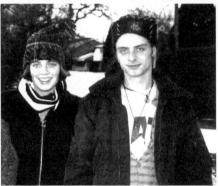

Fig. 2.7 Growth of twins, showing relative heights at different ages.

add something like 20 cm (about 8 in) to their height, mostly because of growth of the trunk, and at the peak of growth velocity at about 14 years of age, they may be growing at the rate of 10 cm/year. Girls gain about 16 cm during the spurt, with a peak velocity about 12 years of age.

The conclusion of the spurt is followed by a rapid slowing of growth: girls reach 98% of their final height by the average age of $16\frac{1}{2}$, whereas boys do not reach the same stage until the age of about $17\frac{3}{4}$; again there is wide variation around the means. Up to the time of the adolescent spurt there is little difference between the average heights of boys and girls, and because the spurt begins earlier in females there is an age at which girls become taller (and heavier) than boys of the same age; in Britain today this age is about 11 years. The balance is redressed by the age of 14, when boys overtake girls in height, although they do not become heavier until some time later (Fig. 2.7).

The control of the adolescent spurt is still not clear, although it is probably affected by genetic influences. For example, a gene called *STST5b* has been found which is active in the male and appears to switch on at puberty, playing a part in the growth spurt. It also has an effect on hair growth, muscle weight, and body fatness.

One consequence of the sexual dimorphism in the timing of the adolescent growth spurt is that girls stop growing earlier than boys who thus have a longer overall time to grow in. Consequently, boys have an average height that is greater than girls at the end of the growing period.

If measurements taken from several children are combined on the same graph, the adolescent spurt is smoothed out and become less dramatic (Fig. 2.6a). This is because the spurt occurs at different times in different children, and, to overcome this difficulty, another way of presenting the information is sometimes used. The peak velocity in each child, irrespective of age, is superimposed on the peaks taken from the others, and this is used as zero time, measurements backwards towards birth being recorded as -1, -2, -3 years, etc., and measurements forwards towards maturity being recorded as $+1$, $+2$, $+3$ years, etc. (Fig. 2.6b).

Humans are the only mammals with such a long quiescent interval before the adolescent spurt, and it has been tentatively suggested that the main reason for this is a need to postpone puberty in order to allow time for the maturation of the more complex human brain. In other words, the delay may be correlated with the fact that human survival depends on learning, which takes time, rather than on instinct, which does not.

It has been found that some children can enter a transitory growth spurt at about the age of 6 or 7 years. This is called the juvenile or mid-growth spurt. Little is known about this spurt as it does not occur in every individual and it is much less than the adolescent spurt.

Although noticeable growth in height stops at about 18 years in the female and 21 in the male, the vertebral column can continue to grow up to about 30 years of age. The total increase in height due to this cause is usually said to be little more than 3–4 mm, and the difficulties of assessing measurements of so small an amount will at once be apparent. Some studies have found that from the age of 19 to the age of 27 the average increase in height for males followed longitudinally was over 2 cm. It is also said that most head measurements continue to increase very slowly up to the age of 60, but the increase from the age of 20 is only about 2–4% of the 20-year values. Growth in height ceases when the growth plates fuse in the vertebral column but this cannot explain how some growth continues beyond attainment of adulthood. What precisely stops growth in height remains unknown, although the influence of the hormones derived from the gonads must be an important factor. Certain cold-blooded animals, such as fish, appear never to stop growing, although they do so at a considerably reduced rate after attaining maturity.

Prediction of adult height

There are a number of situations where there is a need to be able to predict the adult height that a child may attain on completion of growth. Normally, for example, ballerinas should not be taller than 175 cm or smaller than 157 cm with an ideal height of less than 167 cm. As a number of aspiring ballet starlets begin ballet in the early years of childhood, disappointments can be avoided if it could be reliably shown that the adult height of the candidate would be outside the acceptable limits.

Height restrictions used to apply widely in a number of occupations but today these generally have been considerably relaxed. Nurses used to be excluded from training if they were less than 152 cm tall, for the reason that people of this size are not much use at lifting heavy patients. Traditionally, British policemen had to have a height of more than 173 cm and policewomen more than 160 cm, although these standards have been relaxed recently due to recruitment difficulties and other reasons. The armed forces still have minimum height restrictions and there are problems for the very tall who wish to fly aircraft or enter space programmes.

Prediction of likely adult height also has a role in the selection of those wishing to pursue some forms of sporting activities: boys with a predicted adult height of less than 160 cm should be encouraged to think of something other than basketball, and those with a predicted height of 183 cm or over should not train as jockeys. More importantly, excessively tall girls and excessively small boys suffer considerable psychological distress, and if it can be established early on in their growth period that their adult height will render them conspicuous or make it difficult for them to fit into society an attempt can be made to modify future growth before it is too late.

Many parents know that at the age of 2 years a child is approximately half the height it will eventually attain, and some readers may have heard that an estimate of adult height can be obtained by taking the mean of the heights of the parents and adding 5 cm for a boy or subtracting 5 cm for a girl; unfortunately, such simple methods are often extremely inaccurate when applied to an individual.

Analysis of data derived from a sufficient number of children measured longitudinally makes it possible to say what percentage of their final height has been achieved at any given age, and thus to produce a table which will predict, at least roughly, the future height of an individual (Table 2.1). The predictive value of such a table is nil at birth, for the birth length, like the birth weight, is considerably influenced by the environment in the uterus. For example, a baby ultimately destined by its genetic make-up to be tall may measure relatively little at birth if it is premature, one of a multiple birth, or born to a young mother.

But by the second birthday the child should have joined its genetic curve, which is the basic determinant of height, and predictions become possible. A single measurement is of little use, and the child has to be observed over a

Table 2.1 Percentage of mature height attained at different ages

Chronological age (years)	Percentage of eventual height Boys	Girls
1	42.2	44.7
2	49.5	52.8
3	53.8	57.0
4	58.0	61.8
5	61.8	66.2
6	65.2	70.3
7	69.0	74.0
8	72.0	77.5
9	75.0	80.7
10	78.0	84.4
11	81.1	88.4
12	84.2	92.9
13	87.3	96.5
14	91.5	98.3
15	96.1	99.1
16	98.3	99.6
17	99.3	100.0
18	99.8	100.0

The percentages given are derived from a longitudinal study of 150 boys and girls carried out by the University of California (Bayley, N. (1956). *Journal of Pediatrics* **48**, 187–94. Reproduced by kind permission of the author and publishers.)

year or more, because of variations in growth rate with the seasons and other possible causes. If several readings of height are taken in this period, the progress of growth can be compared with standard centile charts. At adolescence these may be confusing if the timing of the adolescent spurt of the patient does not conform to the mean (Fig. 2.6), and it always has to be remembered that the growth curve of an individual does not necessarily run parallel to a centile line. A considerable problem is that the tables refer to normal children, whereas they are perhaps most often used in reference to children who are at least suspected of being abnormal. In such cases considerable caution has to be observed.

Predictions are improved if the heights of the parents are taken into consideration, and Weech's equations are as follows:

$$H_m = 0.545H_2 + 0.544A + either\ 14.84\ \text{(for boys) or } 10.09\ \text{(for girls)}$$

where H_m = height in inches at maturity
H_2 = height in inches at age 2 years
A = mean height in inches of parents

The bone age of a child, and, for girls, the age at which the onset of menstruation occurred are also important factors which can help the accuracy of the calculation. If the child is pre-menarchal, the age at which the mother began to menstruate can be used instead.

In 1975 Tanner and his colleagues calculated for British children a series of equations (the TW2 method) which used the height of the child, its chronological age, its bone age, the time of onset of menstruation, and the average height of the parents. Even this elaborate system could only predict adult height in boys aged 4–12 years to within ±7 cm in 95% of cases. The accuracy improved to ±6 cm at the age of 14. As the 95% range of male height in British adults is ±12.5 cm, such predictions are better than nothing, but they are still disappointingly vague. The figures for girls are similar, except that prediction becomes more accurate earlier; the eventual height of girls of 12 or 13 who have begun menstruating can be predicted to within ±4 cm and ±3 cm respectively.

Box 2.2 TW2 method of prediction of adult height

Adult height prediction is calculated from the child's present height, chronological age and the RUS (radius ulna short) bone age (see p. 104). By use of a series of tables, corrections and coefficients can be applied to the child's data. This is a worked example for a child age 10:

$$H = 1.20 \text{ (height (cm))} - (6.2 \text{ age (years)})$$
$$- (1.0 \text{ RUS bone age (years)}) + 83$$

Full tables with the constants required for each age are given in the *TW2 Atlas*.

Growth in weight

Just as there are difficulties over the apparently simple process of measuring height, so there are problems over obtaining a reliable figure for weight. In the first place, the apparatus may not be consistently accurate. Beam or lever scales are better than the usual bathroom scales, but all must be regularly checked against known weights. The person being weighed must stand still and not sway forward or backward, so altering the pressure on the platform. This requirement is naturally particularly difficult with young children or with babies, who are customarily weighed in a basket arrangement or sling.

As with height, the measurements must be taken at the same time of day, for even with accurate weighing the weight of a healthy person on a constant regimen varies from time to time during the day and also from day to day. In addition, a meal or a full bladder increases weight and a bowel movement decreases it. For these reasons a gain or loss in weight in an adult needs to be

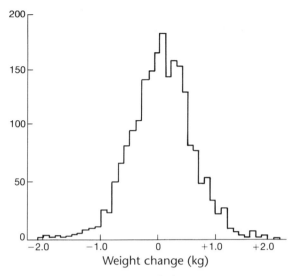

Fig. 2.8 Distributions of alterations in weight (kg) on 2078 occasions on consecutive days in healthy young men. (From Edholm, O. G., Adams, J. M., and Best, T.W. (1974). *Annals of Human Biology*, **1**, 3–12, by kind permission of the editors.)

more than 1 kg to be considered significant (Fig. 2.8).

Growth curves and growth charts

After 280 days of gestation, the new-born baby weighs an average of about 3.4 kg ($7\frac{1}{2}$ lb), with a range of about 2.7–4.5 kg (roughly 6–10 lb). This is something like three thousand million times the weight of the ovum, and gives an idea of the furious growth activity before birth. The maximum growth rate, unlike the maximum rate of growth in height, is not achieved until shortly after birth (Fig. 2.10), but it very soon slackens off markedly, and in the 20 years or so of growth from birth to maturity the birth weight increases by a further factor of only about 20 times—say to an adult weight of 68 kg (150 lb).

The weight at birth is more variable than the length, and reflects the maternal environment more than the heredity of the child. Like body length, it is less when the mother is young, when the baby is premature, and when the mother has become underweight before the pregnancy. Full-term females are on average about 140 g (roughly 5 oz) lighter than full-term males, and a twin weighs on average about 680 g (roughly $1\frac{1}{2}$ lb) less than a singleton; a triplet is about 340 g ($\frac{3}{4}$ lb) lighter than a twin. Small mothers tend to have small babies, irrespective of the size of the father, and mothers in a low socio-economic group have smaller babies than those with a higher rating. The rank of the child in the family is a factor in its birth weight, later children tending to be

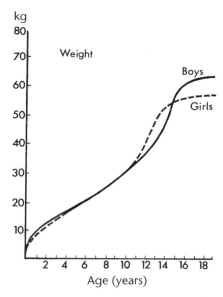

Fig. 2.9 Typical individual weight-attained curves for English boys and girls. (From Tanner, J. M., Whitehouse, R. H., and Takaishi, M. (1966). *Archives of Disease in Childhood*, **41**, 454–71, by kind permission of the authors and the editor.)

somewhat heavier than the first-born. The birth weight is independent of the mother's diet unless there has been severe malnutrition, as the fetus will draw on the mother's tissues for its needs. Women who smoke or drink during pregnancy have smaller babies than those who do not, by about 170 g on the average. Immediately after birth, the diminished intake of fluid leads to a transient loss of about 5% of the birth weight; this loss is usually made good in 10 days or so, and has no connection with the ability of the body to grow.

There is also evidence that with better postnatal care and health in the 1960's and 70's, British babies put on weight in the first few months more rapidly than in the past, possibly due to better diet or feeding. For example, records showed that in 1973, more than 40% of healthy babies in London at the age of 3 months old weighed over 7 kg whereas 20 years earlier fewer than 10% weighed as much at this age.

By the end of the first year the birth weight has approximately tripled, and by the end of the second it has quadrupled. After this it settles down, like the growth in height, to a relatively steady annual increase, which is about 2.25–2.75 kg a year, until the onset of the adolescent spurt (Figs 2.9 and 2.10). During the spurt, boys may add 20 kg to their weight, and girls 16 kg. The peak velocity for the spurt in weight lags behind the peak velocity for height by about 3 months: the child first begins to shoot up, and only later does he/she start to fill out. Similarly, body weight does not reach its adult value until some

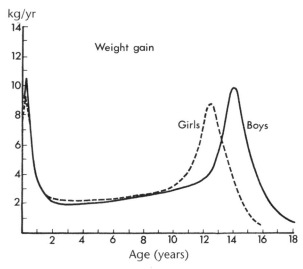

Fig. 2.10 Typical individual velocity curves for weight: English boys and girls. (From Tanner, J. M., Whitehouse, R. H., and Takaishi, M. (1966). *Archives of Disease in Childhood*, **41**, 454–71, by kind permission of the authors and the editor.)

time after adult height has been attained.

Measurements on a large group of children can be combined into a cross-sectional chart showing weight for age in exactly the same way as such charts are constructed for height. Weight for age charts (Figs 2.11 and 2.12) are put to the same sort of use as height for age charts, and are subject to the same limitations. Weight curves of individual children cross-centile lines on the charts more frequently than is the case with height curves. The maximum amount of upward or downward mobility occurs in the first few months of life.

Weight increase is usually taken as a good indicator of satisfactory progress of growth in a child, but variations in the amounts of muscle development and fat deposition make the relationship between height and weight in the growing child a somewhat elastic one. Another factor is the build of the child; mesomorphic and endomorphic children weigh more than ectomorphic children of the same height. In the adult there is a fairly reasonable correlation, and the results of a Scottish survey are shown in Fig. 2.13.

A distinction must be drawn between average and ideal figures of weight for height. The average figures in the United States and Britain are steadily diverging away from the ideal figures laid down by such bodies as the Metropolitan Life Insurance Company in 1943 on the basis of maximum longevity. These figures were continually being revised and are now labelled as 'desirable weights'. The big problem faced by society, particularly in North America and increasingly in Britain is that of obesity. For example, the average weight of males of medium build aged between 25 and 29 years is now

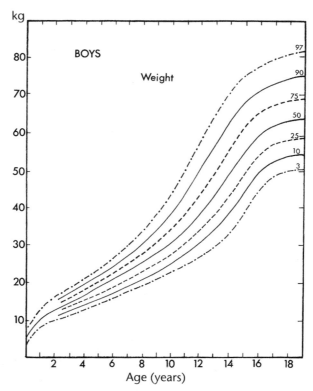

Fig. 2.11 Cross-sectional standards for weight attained at each age: (English boys). The central line represents the mean, or 50th centile. The two dashed lines above and below it represents the 75th and 25th centiles respectively; i.e. 25 per cent of the sample fell below the lower line and 25 per cent above the upper line. Other centile lines are also provided. (Modified from Tanner, J. M., Whitehouse, R. H., and Takaishi, M. (1966). *Archives of Disease in Childhood*, **41**, 454–71, by kind permission of the authors and the editor.)

more than 4.5 kg greater than the insurance company's desirable weight.

The body mass index

The current way of quantifying the status of an individual is to use the 'body mass index' (Quetelet's index), which is defined as the weight in kilograms divided by the square of the height in metres. The rationale of this method is somewhat obscure, but the figures provide a convenient standard which is reasonably independent of height (Fig. 2.14).

Causes of increase in weight

Increases in weight are due to three main factors.

First, muscle weight and size can be increased after puberty by exercise combined with eating a high protein diet that is satisfactory in quantity and

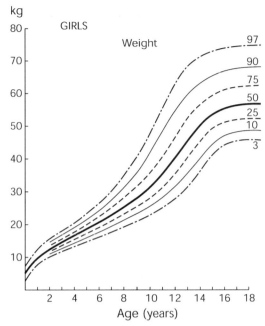

Fig. 2.12 Cross-sectional standards for weight attained at each age: (English girls). Centiles as in Fig. 2.11. (Modified from Tanner, J. M., Whitehouse, R. H., and Takaishi, M. (1966). *Archives of Disease in Childhood*, **41**, 454–71, by kind permission of the authors and the editor.)

quality. There is no increase in the number of fibres, but simply an enlargement of existing ones. However, attempting to increase muscle size in this way before puberty will have a very uncertain outcome.

A second cause of increase in weight is pregnancy, which may well occur before adult weight has been reached. It should be noted that an adolescent girl who has become pregnant will also continue to grow normally throughout the pregnancy.

A normal woman having her first baby in Britain may put on 13–14 kg, although there is a wide range of variation. Four or 5 kg of this is due to the infant, the surrounding fluid, and the placenta, and the greater part of the remainder is accounted for by the growth of the uterus and the breasts. After the uterus has reverted to its resting state, her weight will still be about 5 kg more than it was originally; this is due to the increase in the size of the breasts, and to the stores (mostly of protein and fat) laid down for the feeding of the infant. Some of this weight increase is usually permanent, and the amount of the permanent deposit often increases with each successive child. Women with several children thus tend to be heavier than women with only one or two, and those who are already fat usually put on more weight in pregnancy than those

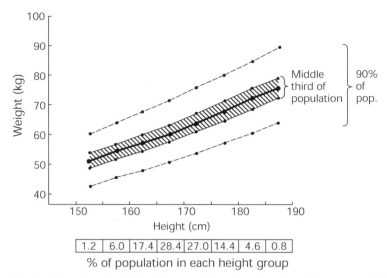

Fig. 2.13 Relationship of adult height to weight. Data from Scottish men aged 18–40 in 1954. (From Sinclair, D. (1976). Growth. In *Textbook of human anatomy*, 2nd edn. (ed. W. J. Hamilton), Macmillan and Co. Ltd., London, by kind permission of the publishers.)

who are initially thin.

Thirdly, it is unfortunately possible to put on weight by eating too much and increasing the fat content of the body. The word 'obese' is defined in the dictionary as 'very fat or fleshy: corpulent', and in medical usage it is now customarily applied to those whose weight exceeds the average for height, age, and sex by 20% or more. Such people are said to have a 'relative weight' of 120, the average being taken as 100. In terms of the body mass index a figure between 20 and 25 is considered acceptable, and obesity is indicated by a figure of 30 or over; gross obesity begins at a figure of 40. However, although the index is appropriate for children and adults, at the time of early puberty it tends to categorize physically advanced adolescents as being overweight.

Obesity

Obesity may develop at any age, and is an increasing health problem. In the United States in 1966 at least 10 per cent of children were thought to be overweight. In Britain, a survey of 300 infants in Worcester in 1972 found that 16.7% were obese and a further 27.7% were over the 90th centile standard for weight. Modern infant foods, coupled with intensive advertising, combine to induce mothers to try to make their children as big and as bouncing as possible, and some years ago it was suspected that in human infants, as in rats, overfeeding in early life could have a permanent effect on fat cellularity and

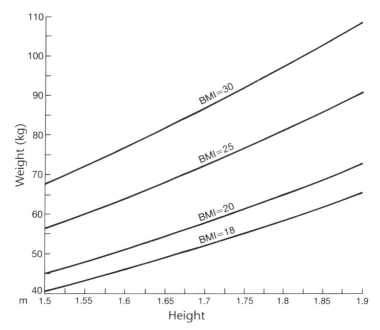

Fig. 2.14 Relationship of adult weight to height. The four curves represent body mass indices of 30, 25, 20, and 18. An index between 20 and 25 is regarded as satisfactory; one over 30 is taken to indicate obesity; and one below 18 to indicate severe undernourishment (see text).

body weight. However, it now seems that most fat babies become normally lean in childhood and adolescence. Nor has the incrimination of early intro-duction of solids to the diet been confirmed as a cause of obesity. The onset of obesity is probably signalled by enlargement of the individual fat cells, which are then stimulated to divide because of their increased size. It has been suggested that this is particularly prone to happen in 'trigger' periods of growth (approximately 0–5 years and 9–13 years of age), but this remains speculative. However, the prevalence of obesity certainly reaches a peak at the age of 11. It then falls until about the age of 20, when it starts to rise again. At the age of 35 more men than women are classified as 'overweight'. The excess fat in men tends to accumulate in the upper abdomen, with the result that they are unkindly described as 'apples'. In women the favoured sites for the fat to collect are the buttocks, hips, and thighs, so bestowing on the victims the equally unkind description of 'pears'. Certain races appear to be genetically prone to obesity, and in the case of the Pima Indians they are mostly 'apples'.

About 40% of British children who are obese at the age of 7 years become obese adults, and if the relative weight at 7 years is 130 or more the risk of becoming an obese adult rises to about 70%. Nevertheless, most obese adolescents do not become obese until after the age of 7. In a survey of children born in 1953 it was found that 9% of adolescent girls and 7% of adolescent boys had a relative weight of 120 or more. Four per cent of girls and 3% of the boys had relative weights of over 130.

There is a high correlation between obesity in the parents and obesity in the children, and this indicates an important genetic factor, as there is no such correlation between the weights of adopted children and their adoptive parents. It is estimated that approximately 70% of children will become obese if both parents are obese, and 50% will do so if one parent is obese; the strongest correlation is between a biological daughter and her mother. If neither parent is affected the risk is only about 10%.

One cannot deposit fat unless sufficient calories are taken in the diet, but many adults and children who eat enormous quantities remain thin, for two people of the same age, sex, body composition, and pattern of activity may differ by up to 40% in their energy expenditure. If the diet contains more calories than the body can use up, particularly if they are supplied by carbohydrate, deposition of fat is inevitable. In adults the advent of middle age is accompanied by a slowing down of general metabolism, but there may be no comparable change in appetite. A lack of exercise then combines with the unnecessary intake of food to cause the accumulation of excess fat, which is one of the problems of so-called civilization.

In rats the lateral part of the hypothalamus contains an 'appetite centre' in which there are high concentrations of certain peptides. Injection of these peptides into the paraventricular nucleus stimulates eating, particularly of carbohydrates and rich food. An interesting, although highly speculative, suggestion is that some such mechanism may operate in humans. However, there is also a genetic component to the equation as it is possible to breed fat mice who put on excessive weight at a rapid rate and become very obese. In this instance, the action of genes controlling the production of a protein called leptin has been identified. Leptin acts to curb the appetite and appears to slow down the metabolism. A defect of a gene in mice called Ob has been found to lead to the absence of the leptin which leads to their obesity. Leptin has been found in humans and is believed to be produced by the hypothalamus. The implications of these findings in humans are still not clear, although they support the concept of genetic factors in controlling obesity.

At all ages, simple greed is only one reason for eating too much; boredom is another, and people who are anxious or unhappy may calm themselves by overeating. A more unusual reason is provided by the professional requirements of Sumo wrestling in Japan. The optimum weight for a Sumo wrestler is about 140 kg, and men training to become wrestlers eat more than 29 000 kJ) daily. They are said to die 10 years younger than the average Japanese, and are prone to diseases of the liver and kidneys.

Competitors in some Olympic events, such as weight-lifting, also find it advantageous to be heavy and so try to put on as much weight as possible. The illegal use of banned anabolic steroid hormones assists the deposition of protein and thus increases the body weight. This can have disastrous results as there have been a number of instances of disease and even death as a consequence of the practice.

It is a hard business fact of the insurance world that dietary excess and obesity in the adult are not good for life expectancy. Successive studies by insurance companies and others in America and Britain have shown that if the relative weight is 120 the mortality rate is about 30% above expectancy. For people with relative weights of 135–145 the rate increases to about 40%, and those who are heavier than this have a mortality more than twice that of the general population. The increased risk is largely due to cardiovascular disease and diabetes mellitus. A body mass index (BMI) of above 29 is suggested as a 'marker' for coronary risk factors, and the least risk of dying within 15 years in American men seems to be when the BMI is about 26, which is slightly above the upper limit of what is usually accepted as 'normal'. In a group of people aged 85 or over in Finland the highest 5-year mortality was in those members with a BMI of under 20 and the lowest in those whose BMI was 30 or over. In very old people it may therefore be that the risk of death does not necessarily increase with the body mass index.

The medical correlates of obesity, which are thought to include such conditions as gallstones, atherosclerosis , and certain cancers, seem to be more strongly related to intra-abdominal fat, as in the 'apples' rather than the 'pears', and the ratio of waist to hip circumference is now regarded as an important clinical measurement, although differences in mortality only become obvious in the highest range of this ratio. The omental fat cells are said to be smaller than the subcutaneous ones, and may differ in their biochemical behaviour.

Diet and anorexia

Today, society has now acquired the new problem of body image and the fear of appearing to be too fat and obese. Major industries have grown up around marketing the best diet to reduce obesity or the most effective bulking agent which makes you feel full-up and no longer want to eat. There is even a demand for drugs which either suppress the appetite or block the absorption of food. The biggest dietary problems affect adolescents, particularly girls, who are frequently driven to dietary extremes by image building in response to advertising where a stick-like figure is perceived as being the norm. Normally, these dietary difficulties appear to resolve themselves without too much risk to growth and development, although it should also be noted that there are the problems of bulimia and anorexia nervosa. In the former, the sufferer induces vomiting after eating a meal whereas in the latter condition, the patient resists eating, and may therefore starve to an extreme degree of emaciation and even death. A BMI of 18 or less is an indication for hospital treatment. Although both conditions are undoubtedly psychiatric in nature and require medical intervention, even here, evidence suggests a genetic basis for the conditions.

In spite of all the propaganda which is developed around diet, in reality it is much more difficult to effect a permanent loss of excess weight than it is to put it on as the body 'defends' a certain plateau of weight once it has become established and mobilizes its metabolism to resist the results of dieting.

Changes in body composition

It is not surprising that there should be variation in measurements of weight. In regard to height, there are only three components to be considered, namely the bones, the cartilages, and a limited amount of connective tissue and skin. In the case of weight, every tissue and organ in the body is involved. In a male, roughly 50% of the adult body weight is due to water located inside the cells, and a further 15% to water in the tissue spaces, making a total of about 65%. In a woman, fat displaces some of the water, so it amounts to only about 52% of the body weight. In the new-born baby, roughly 80% of the body weight is water, 35% intracellular and 45% extracellular. An average adult consumes and excretes about 2000 ml of water daily which amounts to about 5% of the total body fluid. But for an infant the corresponding figures are 600–700 ml, about 20% of the total.

Measurement of body weight at a given moment therefore depends quite considerably on the degree of hydration of the tissues, and this in turn depends on many different influences. For example, women taking contraceptive pills containing oestrogens may gain up to 13 kg in weight through the water-retaining effect of the oestrogen hormones. Conversely, as participants in weight-dependent sports, such as horse-racing or boxing, know, a considerable amount of weight may temporarily be lost by violent sweating following severe exercise or having a sauna. Medically, this is a very dangerous practice as the loss of vital salts is potentially dangerous and also affects the athletic performance of the sportsperson concerned. Patients can also lose water by taking diuretics or purgatives.

Table 2.2 shows the percentage composition by weight of a reference man weighing 70 kg. The figures are derived from the recommendations of the Commission on Radiological Protection, and, like all biological averages, are meaningless when applied to an individual. For example, the range of body fat in apparently normal individuals may be from 12 to 23% of body weight in men and 16 to 28% in women. However, the average figures do give an idea of

Table 2.2 Weight distribution in the adult

Organs or tissues	Percentage of body weight
Muscles	43
Fat	14
Bone and marrow	14
Viscera	12
Connective tissue and skin	9
Blood	8
	100

The figures are averages relating to a male weighing approximately 70 kg.

the contribution made by different tissues and organs to the weight of the adult. But the relative proportions of these tissues vary at different stages of growth. Bone weight remains fairly constant in relation to total weight, but in the infant the muscles account for only about 25% of total weight, whereas in the adult the figure is over 40%. On the other hand, the viscera are relatively heavy in the infant.

Changes in body composition with age

A good deal of effort has recently been put in to trying to find out the composition of the body at different ages. The most obvious method is by direct weighing of viscera, muscles, etc. This can be done in dead bodies, but the results are much more difficult to interpret than might be imagined, partly because the cause of death may itself produce changes in the composition of the body.

Again, it is possible to analyse the composition of an amputated limb, but this result cannot be applied with confidence to an estimate of the composition of the whole body. In a rather different category are the results of chemical determinations of the blood volume, which can be made in intact healthy children.

Radiology has been useful in the estimation of the proportions of fat and muscle in the limbs. A soft-tissue radiograph will show the relative widths of the shadows cast by the bone and the muscle, and the amount of fat can be obtained from the distance between the outer border of the muscle shadow and the skin.

Formulae exist by which measurements made at selected places can be transformed into estimates of the proportions of these tissues in the whole body.

Another way of determining the amount of fat in the body is to measure with special callipers the width of skin folds pinched up at different places. Two sites frequently used are on the back of the arm over the triceps muscle and on the back of the trunk below the angle of the scapula; reference standards exist for the dimensions of the skinfolds at different ages. Estimates of total body fat based on such measurements, like those derived from radiography, are little more than informed guesses, since there is no reliable correlation between subcutaneous fat and the amount of fat in the abdominal cavity. But both methods do yield a satisfactory estimate of subcutaneous fat, and the thickness of the triceps skinfold correlates well with body density (obtained by an underwater weighing technique); it is now used as an index of total body fat. Other ways of determining this quantity are still less direct and of uncertain accuracy. For example, the total body water can be measured and from this the 'lean body mass' can be calculated. This is then subtracted from the total body mass to give a figure representing the total body fat. Electrical impedance testing and absorption of near-infrared light by the arm have been used, and intra-abdominal fat has been assessed by computed tomography.

Finally, it is possible to calculate the total amount of muscle in the body very roughly by measuring the power of a limited group of muscles, such as those of the upper limb. Similar caution must be observed in relating such measurements to the total musculature, but direct comparisons between individuals can be made without objection.

The merits of size

Limitations are imposed on the size range of the human body, and we could never be as large as an elephant without undergoing drastic internal reconstruction. It was Galileo who pointed out that 'Nature cannot construct an animal beyond a certain size, while retaining the proportions and employing the materials which suffice in the case of a smaller structure.' The reason for this is to be found in the same laws that limit the size of cells. The volume of similar bodies, and hence their weight, increases with the cube of the linear dimensions: a guinea-pig 12.5 cm long is nearly twice as heavy as one 10 cm long. At the same time, the cross-sectional area of the bones which support this weight only increases with the square of the linear dimensions.

J. B. S. Haldane once calculated that the giants in the illustrations in his copy of the Pilgrim's Progress must have been about 18 m tall. These giants would weigh about 1000 times as much as a normal human, but the cross-section of their bones would be only 100 times greater. Hence every square centimetre of bone in the giant would have to support 10 times the weight borne by a square centimetre of bone in a normal human. But this is just about the breaking strain of human bone, and Haldane concluded that the giants would break their thighs with every step they took, unless some radical alterations had been made in their internal construction, and different material substituted for bone.

Another mechanical difficulty is caused by the increased bending moments to which bone is subjected in a large animal. The amount of sag of a beam under its own weight varies as the square of the length of the beam, and in consequence the limbs, if they are to avoid breaking, must become thicker and shorter as the animal increases in size. Merely to increase the linear dimensions of human beings is therefore not possible beyond a certain point, for their existence would become most precarious.

In mythology, giants were viewed as possessing enormous strength. The strength of a muscle depends on two main factors, the number of fibres which can be brought to bear, and the pull exerted by each fibre. The number of fibres pulling depends on the cross-section of the muscle, and this, like that of the bones, increases with the square of the linear dimensions. But the weight which the muscles have to move increases with the cube of the same dimensions, so that on this account a very large person would be relatively more feeble than one of normal size. However, the pull of each fibre depends up to a point on the number of contractile units along its length, and the total number of these varies with the volume of the muscle, which increases with the cube of the linear dimensions. Large people are not, therefore, at so great a disadvantage as might be expected, and power more or less keeps pace with body size.

The surface area of the body, like the cross-section of the bones, only increases as the square of the linear dimensions. This means that if all dimensions of one body are 10% greater than those of another body of the same shape, the larger body has 33% more weight, but only 21% more surface area. The rate at which heat is lost to the environment depends on the surface area exposed, and food intake and oxygen consumption must balance the loss of heat, otherwise death would ensue. A large person therefore needs less food per unit of weight than a small person does to keep warm, and small people, like infants, are more vulnerable in situations where excessive heat loss is liable to occur, such as exposure to extreme cold.

In conformity with this principle it was once postulated that the largest animals should be found in cold climates, and the smallest in the tropics, but, although the proponents of this idea could point to polar bears and whales, the elephants and other large tropical animals such as the hippopotamus and the rhinoceros were conveniently forgotten. It was later urged that within a given genus the species enlarged in size as one progressed away from the tropics. There was more to commend this argument, but there are exceptions. For example, otters tend to become smaller as their geographical range becomes colder.

The relation of human size to climate will be discussed in Chapter 8, but it may be said here that any systematic effect of this kind is outweighed by genetic influences and other factors such as diet. There is, however, some evidence that body shape may be determined in part by climatic surroundings. It is interesting to examine the devices which the larger animals have been obliged to adopt in order to increase the area of vitally important surfaces to correspond with the increased weight, and hence increased metabolic activity, of the body. The absorptive mucous membrane of the small intestine, for example, is thrown into circular folds, upon each of which have been developed large numbers of finger-like villi (the same device is used in the household bath-towel). The lungs have developed an enormous surface area by spreading their capillaries out on the walls of the alveoli; the cortex of the brain has been thrown into folds. These modifications parallel on the gross scale the changes in shape which individual cells may adopt in order to avoid the restrictions imposed by the surface/volume ratio, and, like the microscopic modifications, cannot be effective beyond a certain point.

Short stature and gigantism

Within the human population, a range of different mechanisms must act together towards imposing regulation on the average size of individuals within society and set the limits to what is possible without major changes being required to the underlying body structure. This limit has developed as the human frame has evolved over the last few million years from our ancestors. What we now require is a determination of what these limits are and this raises difficulties for the human biologist.

It is fairly straightforward to obtain the average height and weight for any given population using standard surveying techniques and within such a sample, there are bound to be a few individuals who are small or are large. It is the extreme of human size for which it is difficult to obtain accurate actual measurements.

These extremes of excessive or minimal height have always been exploited within society either as entertainment, such as those who employ their short stature or gigantism for the show, circus, cinema, or theatre, or in mythology and stories passed down as the oral tradition of any race of people or tribe. The tale of David and Goliath is such a tale and there are many mythical giants described in Nordic legends. Wild exaggerations of size are also common, with some giants having an impossible size, such as Finn MacCool, who threw the Isle of Man across from Ireland, leaving behind Lough Neagh, the hole from which it was torn.

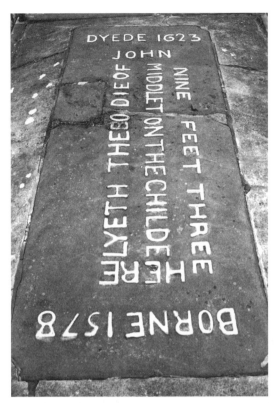

Fig. 2.15 The tomb of John Middleton, known as Childe of Hale, in Hale churchyard, Cheshire. The inscription reads Here lyeth the bodie of John Middleton, the Childe. Nine feet three. Born 1578 Dyede 1623. Exhumation of the tomb in 1768 revealed a femur which measured 86 cm in length.

Patrick Byrne, a real Irish 'giant', was thought during his life to be very much taller than the 231 cm which his skeleton was found to measure when John Hunter, the famous surgeon, succeeded in obtaining it for investigation after many difficulties. John Middleton, known as the Childe of Hale, was born in 1578 in Hale near Liverpool and was of normal size until his adolescence when he then grew to reach 280 cm. When his tomb was opened, large bones were found in it but no actual measurements seem to survive. People over 230 cm in height are undeniably rare, but Arey cites a height of 289 cm as the known extreme. The tallest man of whom there are authentic measurements was probably Robert Wadlow, an American born in 1918, who at his death at the age of 22 measured 272 cm.

The causes of most cases of giantism are due to disorders of the pituitary gland while the causes of short stature are much more variable. Most frequently they are due to a skeletal dysplasia such as achondroplasia (which may be genetically determined) but they can also be a consequence of pituitary deficiency. Perhaps the most famous case of short stature was General Tom Thumb, who was exploited by the Circus owner Barnum, but many smaller examples of short stature have been recorded, including an individual who was 48 cm tall at the age of 18 years and weighed only 5.45 kg. There were two siblings, one of whom measured 56 cm and the other 84 cm; the father was 188 cm in height and the mother 168 cm. Gul Mohammed, who lived in New Delhi, India, died in 1997 and measured only 57 cm in height.

Even if we are satisfied to have obtained an estimate of the probable extremes of the range of human size, there will still remain the problem (so common in all biological measurements) of defining the limits of what may be considered 'normal' or 'abnormal'. In Africa, Dinka women, for example, would be considered extremely if not abnormally tall in Britain, whereas a pygmy would be viewed as suffering from short stature. But when is a member of a specified race to be considered a giant or having short stature? However the categorization is made, there is always an overlap zone with the spectrum of normality when an individual may be thought of as either a very small 'normal' or having short stature or a very large 'normal' or giant. Consequently, the spectrum of normality will include many people who are large and others who are small, each bringing with it advantages and disadvantages for the individual.

The problems of extremes of size

Much human sport has developed around considerations of large or small size and shape with such qualities frequently determining the type of activity an individual sportsperson will engage in and excel. For example, large individuals will tend to be best suited for basket-ball and net-ball while heavy build and weight will favour the members of the scrum in a rugby team.

However, there are drawbacks to being excessively large which derive from the fact that large people have not only a greater inertia, but also a greater momentum than smaller ones; it follows that as a rule small people have greater agility. As D'Arcy Thompson said: 'Among animals we shall see, without the help of mathematics or of physics, how small birds and beasts are quick and agile, and how slower and sedater movements come with larger size, and how exaggerated bulk brings with it a certain clumsiness, a certain inefficiency, an element of risk and hazard, a preponderance of disadvantage.'

Nevertheless, the maximal speed of which a large person is capable is very similar to the maximal speed of a small person. A.V. Hill. who investigated this problem, pointed out that 'if one animal is 1000 times as heavy as another, its linear dimensions will be 10 times as great, it will take 10 times as long for one movement, but since that movement is 10 times as great, its linear speed over the ground will be the same'. Large animals actually have an advantage in staying power: Hill calculated that it would take 10 times as long for the larger animal to become exhausted as it would for the smaller animal when both were exerting a maximal effort. To quote D'Arcy Thompson again: 'in the Oxford and Cambridge boat race it is prudent and judicious to bet on the heavier crew.'

There are specific difficulties about being large in our present civilization. Although tall people can see over hedges and are better off in a crowd when they can see over others, they have enormous trouble with the apparatus of everyday life. Problems then arise in driving cars and other vehicles where the designer created a seating position for a normal frame which cannot accommodate the tall person. This used to be a major problem for tall Western people fitting into Japanese and other Asian cars designed for populations where the average adult size is smaller. Computer users need to adopt comfortable positions to use their equipment and this can be difficult for a tall person if their seat cannot adjust enough when the desk is too low, resulting in their craning their neck to view their VDU. Tall women can still encounter great difficulty in obtaining ready-to-wear clothes and shoes, although this may be less of a problem today than in the past. Whereas the seating in cars, cinemas, schools, and other public places was often atrociously designed, awareness of the size range and the problems of the taller person is now being addressed by the design industry through wider application of anthropometry and ergonomics.

It is the science of ergonomics which has gone a long way towards addressing the ethnic and size diversity that occurs in humankind and helps to meet the problems of the taller person. It is an important component of design for everyday living, as mankind is at present still increasing in height and weight. This process is called secular change and is having marked effects in races who have traditionally been viewed as small, such as in Japan and China.

It is also possible that the composition of the human body may eventually alter in response to the increase in size. It is a general principle of biology that in all except the simplest organisms growth of the various components of the body is differential, so that all parts of the body do not increase proportionately. If an increase in the size of a given animal occurs in the course of evolution, it is common for differential growth to produce structural and functional changes in its organs and tissues, and, indeed, this seems to be one of the basic methods of natural selection. The changes which might occur in the human body in response to an increase in size are impossible to predict, and afford an interesting field for writers of science fiction.

Resource

A useful source of information is the Internet.

The metropolitan Life (USA) figures for height and ideal weight can be found at http://www.room42.com/nutrition/metlife.html

Fitness and health. Go and ask Alice at:

http://www.columbia.edu/cu/healthwise/Cat3.html

3   Growth of tissues

It is not growing like a tree
In bulk, doth make men better be
Johnson

Connective tissue

The connective tissues in the body contribute substantially to the bulk of the body, being found in association with all tissues and organs. Relatively little is known about its growth after the embryonic period, although study of the deposition of collagen fibres from work on tendons has shown us some of the processes involved. In baby animals, tendons are relatively cellular, but as growth proceeds the cellular content diminishes, and in adult tendon there are very few cells in comparison with the number of fibres. The thickness of a tendon (and thus the number of collagen fibres developed in it) appears to depend on the severity and duration of the stresses to which it is subjected. There is no strict relationship between the size of a muscle and the size of its tendon, and if a muscle belly is removed from a baby animal, leaving the tendon behind, the tendon, which is subjected only to incidental passive tensions during movement of adjacent muscles, may reach as much as 85% of its normal adult diameter. But if the incidental movements are eliminated as far as possible by fixing the adjacent joints, the isolated tendon may not grow beyond its size at operation. Collagen fibres seem to be laid down in connective tissue along the lines of stress to which the tissue is subjected, and at first they have a narrow size range, which broadens at maturity. It is probable that the amount of collagen in any given situation depends on the magnitude of the local stresses. In a healing wound it has been shown that the directional posture adopted by the fibroblasts is determined by the tensional forces acting on the wound. Such a mechanism also accounts for the development of the retention bands which bind down tendons, the pulleys which alter their direction of action, and the ligaments which restrain excessive movements.

As already stated, the connective tissues make a substantial contribution to the weight of the body. The subcutaneous tissue alone accounts for as much as a quarter of the birth weight, and in the adult it contributes 6–7% of the total weight in males and almost double this in females. The importance of connective tissue in relation to height is much less, and only two regions are involved, the scalp and the heel. The scalp need not detain us, although it does appear to participate in the adolescent spurt, but the fibrofatty pad of the heel, together with the specially thickened skin in this region, may constitute a layer of 2 cm or more in depth. Virtually nothing is known about the development or growth of such pads.

At birth the bursae under tendons and muscles are well developed, but those under the skin may or may not be present.

Body fat

There was once some argument as to whether fat 'grows' in the same sense as the other tissues. The fat of the body is contained in connective tissue cells which are initially indistinguishable from fibroblasts, and it was thus maintained that fat is merely a chemical deposit taken up by connective tissue cells in the course of their life, and that there are no such things as 'fat cells' or 'adipose tissue'. But fat does not occur in all parts of the body: the subcutaneous tissue of the eyelids, the external ear, the nose, the back of the hand, and the scrotum contain very little fat indeed. On the other hand, fat is stored in the subcutaneous tissue elsewhere, and in the omenta of the peritoneum. This has been taken to mean that fat cells compose a specific kind of connective tissue with a definite distribution, and the conclusion is supported by the fact that connective tissue taken from a site where fat normally accumulates still forms adipose tissue if transplanted to another site which is normally fat-free.

It is possible to determine the number and size of the fat cells ('adipocytes') in a sample of fat. In rats the number increases in the early stages of growth, and can be permanently increased by overfeeding at this stage. However, after the animal has attained skeletal maturity (about 15 weeks of age) there is no further increase in number, and fat deposits grow purely by cellular enlargement. If the rat is now starved, or if overfeeding is continued, the number of adipocytes remains unchanged but the size of the individual fat cells alters.

But even if fat is a deposit in a specific kind of tissue, it is still in rather a different category from muscle, bone, etc., for the fat deposits in the body are largely a means of storing energy, and at any stage during growth they can come and go according to the nutrition of the individual. Not all stores of fat are equally labile. Thus, fat in the subcutaneous tissue and in the omenta is readily drawn upon in case of need, but other deposits, such as those in close relation to viscera like the heart and kidneys, are kept in being even in quite severe malnutrition.

Fat appears in the subcutaneous tissue about the sixth month of fetal life, and is plentiful in this situation in the new-born baby, probably as an insulation against cooling. It accounts for about 25% of the total weight of the infant. Characteristic pads of fat at the inner sides of the soles of the feet may give the impression that the baby is flat-footed; they disappear later. A suctorial pad of fat in the cheek is supposed to aid in sucking, although the mechanism is speculative. The infant has little fat in several places where it is prominent in the adult; the omenta are small and undeveloped, and there is not much fat round the kidneys.

On the other hand, there is an accumulation of brown fat in the neck, round the kidneys and in the region of the scapulae; unlike ordinary fat, this tissue has a rich nerve and blood supply, and when the body is exposed to cold it can be rapidly hydrolysed and oxidized in a reaction which produces much heat. In rats it has an important protective role in temperature regulation, and this is emphasized by the fact that it is selectively spared in malnutrition. It has also been suggested that it may play a part in regulating weight by expending energy. For a time it was thought to play a similar part in the human body, but its importance in humans is now believed to be slight. During the first 10 years of life the human brown fat continues to be widely distributed, but thereafter it gradually disappears from most areas, although it persists, even into old age, round the kidneys, the adrenals, and the aorta.

Both sexes have equal amounts of fat at birth, and the fat content of the body increases considerably between birth and the age of 6 months, but the rate of increase rapidly falls off in the last 6 months of the first year. After this the fat content actually decreases till the age of 6 or 8 years, by which time the thickness of the subcutaneous tissue is approximately half what it was at the age of 1 year. The decrease is less in girls than in boys, so that after 1 year of age girls are fatter than boys of the same age.

Subsequently, the body fat begins to increase again, and many children put on excess fat just before the adolescent spurt; this may lead to emotional problems. During the male spurt the fat on the limbs decreases, and is not gained back until the late twenties. In girls there is no such decrease, although there may be a temporary interruption of the increase. In both sexes fat on the trunk continues to increase fairly steadily, but in girls additional fat is laid down in the secondary sexual distribution (Fig. 3.1). This means that at puberty a girl has roughly about twice as much fat as a boy.

More recently, it has been found that the biochemical composition of the body fat is altering with the discovery that the proportion of stearic and oleic acids is falling while the proportion of linoleic acid is rising. This is undoubtedly a consequence of the increased intake of vegetable fats associated with a decreased consumption of red meat and animal fat as it is perceived that such fat is healthier and may protect the body from cardiovascular disease. There is some concern that this may lead to other new long-term risks due to the excessive quantity of these fats in the body, but this remains unclear and controversial.

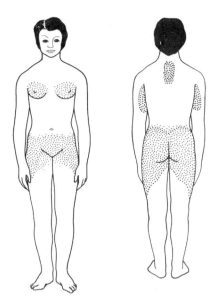

Fig. 3.1 Sites of deposition of fat in the female body at puberty.

Skin

The skin at birth is relatively thin and easily damaged; it accounts for about 4% of the total body weight in the new-born, and about 6% in the adult. As there are about $800\,\text{cm}^2$ of skin per kilogram of body weight in the infant and only about $300\,\text{cm}^2$ in the adult, the disparity in thickness is greater than these percentages suggest at first sight. Sebaceous glands are present before birth, and their secretion is the main constituent of the vernix caseosa, a cheesy material covering the surface of the new-born baby and filling the external auditory meati. The sebaceous glands are relatively inactive for some time after birth, and they grow very rapidly during the adolescent spurt, at which time blackheads, pimples, and acne are rife. These are associated with the profound hormonal changes which occur at puberty; eunuchs do not suffer from acne.

The sweat glands in the new-born baby are immature and function poorly; this is important because of the effect on the regulation of the body temperature. They reach the adult level of function by about the age of 2 years.

In the later stages of fetal life there is a generalized covering of delicate hairs known as the lanugo, but these are mostly lost before birth, and after a few weeks those that remain are replaced by secondary hairs, also fine, known as the vellus. The persistent lanugo hairs on the scalp and eyebrows are shed after a few months and replaced by thicker 'terminal' hairs. At adolescence the coarse secondary sexual hair appears, under the influence of the secretions of the gonads.

No new hair follicles are formed after birth, except in response to local trauma, and the successive changes in the type of hair occur in the same pre-existing follicle. The transition from vellus to terminal hairs may be abrupt or gradual; in the latter case successive generations of hairs in the same follicle form a transition. Each follicle is specific for its own type of terminal hair, and will continue to produce it if transplanted elsewhere; thus, hair from the scalp will not change its character if transplanted to the pubic region and vice versa. Occasionally, the hair pattern can be disturbed by certain follicles producing a type of hair inappropriate to the age and sex of the patient.

The skin and its appendages are a convenient site in which to observe growth in the adult, and further details will be given in Chapter 9.

Muscle and tendon

The composition of muscle varies with age; in the fetus it contains a great deal of water and much intercellular matrix, but after birth both are considerably reduced as the cells grow in size by accumulating cytoplasm. There is curiously little information on the numbers of fibres in a given muscle at different ages. In 1898, counts made on the human sartorius muscle indicated that there is no multiplication of fibres in this muscle after the fourth or fifth month of fetal life, and that the subsequent increase in size is due to enlargement of the existing fibres. It is generally agreed that this finding also applies to the other muscles of the human body, although in rats and mice the number of fibres in a given muscle may increase with age in the period immediately after birth. In contrast to the fibres, muscle fibrils remain constant in diameter as the muscle grows, and their number increases. They grow in length at their ends. The growth of the connective tissue components of a muscle is maximal in the vicinity of the junction of the tendon with the muscle. Mitotic figures in skeletal muscle after birth do not occur within the muscle fibres, but in the undifferentiated cells outside them. These 'satellite' cells appear early in development, and their nuclei account for 5–10% of the total number in the muscle. They multiply to reproduce their kind and also to form muscle cells, which fuse together to increase the length of the muscle fibre. There may be two distinct populations of satellite cells, one which perpetuates the race of satellite cells and the other which produces new muscle cells.

The total mass of muscle in the body can be estimated from the amount of creatinine excreted in the urine, as the conversion of creatine to creatinine takes place only in muscle. The number of nuclei in a known volume of muscle removed at biopsy can be estimated by finding the amount of deoxyribonucleic acid (DNA) it contains, as the amount of DNA per nucleus is constant. From these two sets of figures the number of muscle nuclei in the body can be obtained. It has been found that in the gluteal muscles of boys the number increases 14-fold between birth and maturity; in girls the increase is 10-fold. The diameter of the muscle fibres reaches a maximum in girls about the age of 10, and not until about the age of 14 do the boys catch up. Although it seems clear that the increase in length of muscle fibres is paralleled by an increase in the number of nuclei in the fibres, the question regarding a possible increase in the number of muscle fibres remains unsolved.

A potent stimulus to the growth of a muscle is the separation of its attachments as the skeleton grows, and it has been suggested that the length of a muscle fibre is the direct consequence of the range of movement it is called upon to perform. Common sense would certainly support this, for if the fibres were too short they would rupture under the strain of a full movement, and if they were too long they could not exercise their full potential for contraction. The stimulus for the formation of a tendon is probably the pull of the muscle rudiment on undifferentiated connective tissue, and certainly repair of a tendon from which a segment has been removed does not occur if the muscle is prevented from exercising tension on the cut tendon.

If the tibialis anterior of an experimental animal is released from the extensor retinaculum, thus making the distance between the bony attachments of the muscle shorter, the growth of the tendon is retarded. But because the muscle fibres now have to contract over a greater range in order to produce the same amount of movement at the ankle joint, there is an actual increase in the length of the muscle belly. Interestingly, patients who damage their Achilles tendon (tendo calcaneus) often find their calf muscle never regains its former size, suggesting muscle growth is stimulated by tendon length or perhaps nerve factors as yet not identified.

Replacement of muscle by tendon ('tendinification') sometimes appears to be the result of limitation of movement. In animals such as the baboon, the coccygeus passes from the ischial spine to the mobile coccygeal vertebrae, and is a fleshy muscle throughout; in humans, where the upper part of the muscle is attached to the immovable sacrum, this portion is converted into fibrous tissue.

If the normal opponents of a muscle are paralysed, the muscle fails to grow properly, and the full development of a muscle is probably dependent on the progressive rise in the tension exerted on it by its antagonists.

Many of the fibres in the muscles of baby laboratory animals are relatively rich in the enzyme myosin-ATPase, which enables them to contract rapidly. As the animal grows, the proportion of such fibres falls, particularly in the postural muscles, which have to maintain the increasing body weight against gravity for progressively longer periods. Curiously, the proportion of fast fibres rises again in old age, at least in some muscles. It has not yet been established whether the relative proportions of these kinds of fibres in human muscles change between childhood and adult life.

The growth of muscle is a big factor in the adolescent spurt in weight.

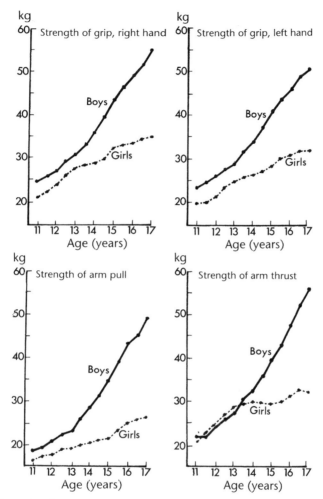

Fig. 3.2 Strength of grip, arm pull, and arm thrust. Mixed longitudinal data. Note the divergence of the curves for boys away from the curves for girls at the time of the adolescent spurt. (From Tanner, J. M. (1962). *Growth at adolescence* (2nd edn). Blackwell Scientific Publications Ltd., Oxford, by kind permission of the author and publishers.)

Before the time of the adolescent spurt, the strength of boys and girls shows little difference, but after it males have the advantage (Fig. 3.2). The curve for the increase in strength lags about a year behind the curve for the increase in body weight; hence there is a limited sense in which children may be said to 'outgrow their strength'. Maximal muscular strength is usually attained between 25 and 30 years of age, and after this there is a gradual and small falling off in both the speed and power of contraction. After 50, the muscles become considerably reduced in size.

The muscles of the head, trunk, and upper limbs are relatively heavier in the infant because of the poor development of the lower limbs; in the adult about 55% of the weight of the musculature is accounted for by the lower limb muscles. The respiratory muscles and those of facial expression are well developed at birth to provide for the vital functions of breathing and sucking, but others, such as the levator ani, have been described by Crelin as having 'the consistency of moist tissue paper'. The weight of the musculature can be increased, in both children and adults, by exercise.

A good deal less is known about visceral and cardiac muscle than is known about somatic muscle. The cells of visceral muscle increase both in number and in size, but the latter process is the more important; it has been calculated that visceral muscle can increase in bulk by a factor of eight times merely by the enlargement of its fibres. Cardiac muscle also increases in bulk by enlargement of existing fibres, a condition frequently observed in older people who suffer from medical conditions such as heart failure.

Nervous tissue

Research has shown that by the end of the fifth month of pregnancy, all nerve cells have been formed within the nervous system, especially within the cerebral cortex. Subsequent growth is therefore dependent on the increase in growth of the specialized supportive cell tissues and the increase in size of existing cell bodies. Nerve growth factors support this growth and development. Ramification and myelination of the axon processes of nerve cells ensures more and more complex connections and assemblies occur between them. This process is also accompanied by the elimination and death of whole populations of neurones by the process of naturally occurring cell death. This consequential cell death is due to cells competing for life-sustaining nutrients called trophic factors which are supplied in limited quantities by target cells. These trophic factors are part of a large family of proteins called neurotrophins which, with nerve growth factors, are responsible for maintaining the various links between nerve cells in the brain.

Growth of the nervous system is accompanied by a continual remodelling of connections between cells which are contstantly establishing and losing links every second. There is a period during early growth when there is considerable plasticity in this remodelling but after a critical period, it appears that the central nervous system loses this ability to regrow and realign. Recently, it has been shown that neurotrophins are probably also responsible for inhibiting new growth of cells in the central nervous system if it is damaged after the critical period. This is an exciting area of research as certain neurotrophins have been demonstrated to remove inhibitions to regrowth in damaged parts of the central nervous system. It holds out great prospects for the treating of victims of strokes and spinal cord injury. They are also thought to play a major part in the generation of pain and are currently an area of interest to those researching pain relief.

Once formed, a nerve cell can increase in mass up to 200 000 times, most of the addition being to the processes of the cell, each of which may come to contain as much as a thousand times the amount of material contained in the cell body. The diameter of the myelinated nerve fibres in peripheral nerve trunks increases considerably during growth, and the nerve cell is rich in ribonucleic acid (RNA), which is used for the energy-expensive task of forming cytoplasm to be pushed outwards into these fibres. In tissue culture the growth of nerve cells in size and in number is specifically stimulated by nerve growth factors, which can be isolated from a number of curious places, such as the salivary glands of mice.

Myelination (Fig. 3.3) is a progressive process which is far from complete at birth. It commences in the second trimester of pregnancy in the peripheral nerves where the motor nerves myelinate before the sensory ones. In contrast, in the brain and spinal cord, the process begins in the sensory nerves before the motor nerves. The first fibres to myelinate have very different diameters, and there seems to be no critical size or range of sizes at which myelination begins. In general, the larger the fibre, the thicker its myelin sheath, but this association is not a regular one. As the length of the myelinated fibres

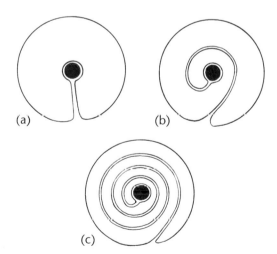

Fig. 3.3 Scheme of the process of myelination. (a) Cross-section of a nerve fibre embedded in the cytoplasm of a Schwann cell. The gutter along which the fibre was engulfed by the Schwann cell still remains open to the surface. (b) The Schwann cell and the fibre rotate relative to each other, so winding the adjacent surfaces of the Schwann cell membrane round the fibre. (c) A further stage of the winding process, showing several double layers of membrane surrounding the fibre. These tightly wound wrappings fuse together to form the myeline sheath of the fibre.

increases, the total number of nodes of Ranvier appears to remain constant, and it follows that the length of the internodal segments increases with growth. After a fibre has been surrounded with myelin, it continues to require further myelination on account of growth both in length and in diameter. The spiral winding mechanism of myelination shown in Fig. 3.3 cannot apply in the central nervous system, where myelination is effected by the connective tissue oligodendrocytes, as a single oligodendrocyte can form myelin sheaths round a number of separate fibres simultaneously.

Cartilage and bone

The skeleton contributes about 14% to the weight of the adult body, and, along with the fibrocartilaginous intervertebral discs, some 97–98% of the total height. (The remaining 2–3% is due to the thickness of the scalp and the fibrofatty pad of the heel, together with the thickness of the articular cartilages in the lower limb and in the atlanto-occipital joint.)

A great deal more is known about the growth of human bone than about the growth of any other human tissue, because of the accessibility of bone to investigation in the living person by means of radiology. It is therefore possible to discuss the processes involved in some detail.

Formation and growth of cartilage

Towards the end of the first month of fetal life the embryonic connective tissue in the region of the future skeleton begins to show signs of differentiation. The primitive cells become more closely packed, and lose the processes which up to now have radiated from them. Later they begin to lay down a matrix rich in chondroitin sulphate (cartilage is about 70% water, and, of the residue, 80% is collagen and sulphated polysaccharides), and this gradually separates the cells from each other again. The cells surrounding the developing cartilage begin to form two layers: in the outer one they differentiate into fibroblasts, and coincident with this collagen is laid down. The cells of the inner layer remain more or less undifferentiated and capable of division to produce cartilage cells. The two layers together are called the perichondrium.

The newly formed cartilage grows larger in two ways, by interstitial and by appositional growth. Interstitial growth occurs because the cells in the centre of the developing mass do not immediately lose their power to divide. The new cells which they form join with the older ones in laying down more and more matrix, and the whole tissue grows as dough does in bread-making.

Obviously, this process depends on the matrix being pliable, and after a short while it becomes too rigid for much interstitial growth to occur; the second mechanism, appositional growth, then predominates.

In this process the cells of the deeper layer of the perichondrium divide: some of the offspring remain as stem cells, and others differentiate, so that more and more cartilage is laid down on the surface of the existing mass. The differentiated cells surround themselves with matrix in the usual way, and are in turn overlaid by successive new layers so that they gradually sink into the depths. As the mass increases in size, the surface area of the perichondrium expands to cover it, and an increasing number of stem cells is therefore required.

Ossification

During the second month of fetal life, bone formation begins. In a few bones, such as the clavicle and the bones of the vault of the skull, ossification begins directly in the connective tissue of the embryo, and such bones are said to be ossified 'in membrane'. The remaining bones of the skeleton are ossified 'in cartilage', which means that the same sort of process takes place after the connective tissue has become converted into a sort of cartilaginous template: the only difference is that cartilage bones have to go through this extra stage.

The points at which bone formation begins are known as 'primary centres' of ossification, and these centres appear in different bones at different times, the first usually being either the mandible or the clavicle, at about the fifth week of fetal life. In a membrane bone, the first sign of ossification is the penetration of a blood vessel to the spot, bringing with it specialized cells called osteoblasts and osteoclasts. Around the osteoblasts, which are modified fibroblasts, collagen fibres are deposited, and on these fibres calcium salts and other inorganic salts accumulate. The osteoclasts, which are large multinucleated cells derived from the bone marrow stem cells, have the task of shaping the growing bone tissue by removing unwanted material. There has been a great deal of controversy about the exact methods employed by the osteoblasts and osteoclasts, and the matter is too complicated to go into in a book of this size. However, it is generally accepted that osteoblasts are concerned with bone deposition and osteoclasts with its removal.

The activities of the two types of cell are related in some manner, perhaps by a local chemical mechanism. Together they are grouped in 'basic multicellular units' which also contain mononuclear cells. It is believed that the osteoblasts are in control of these units and dictate the behaviour of the other cells. On the surface of bones the osteoblasts and osteoclasts work shifts; a period of absorption is followed by a period of new bone deposition.

In the primary centre of a cartilage bone, the first sign of ossification is that the cartilage cells swell up, and arrange themselves in columns. At the same time calcium salts are deposited in the matrix of the cartilage, converting it into 'calcified cartilage'. A blood vessel now grows into the region from the

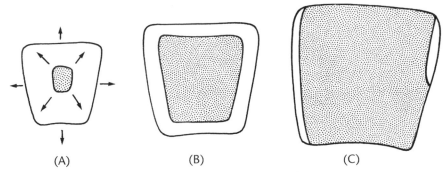

Fig. 3.4 Growth of short bone. (A) The core of newly formed bone in the centre of the cartilaginous 'model' increases in size at the expense of the cartilage. At the same time the cartilaginous model itself grows by activity of the perichondrium. (B) Growth of new bone proceeds faster than growth of cartilage, so that a greater proportion of the developing structure is composed of bone. (C) Bone formation has outstipped cartilage formation and the whole structure is now composed of bone with the exception of a large cartilaginous articular facet on one surface and a smaller one on the opposite surface. This is the adult state for this particular bone, and growth now ceases.

perichondrium, bringing with it osteoblasts and osteoclasts as in the case of membrane bones. The osteoclasts remove some of the calcified cartilage, collagen fibres appear round the osteoblasts, and gradually the calcified cartilage is replaced by true bone.

Growth of short bones

The subsequent growth of a short bone such as one of the cuneiform bones of the foot can be illustrated by a diagram (Fig. 3.4). In the centre of the cartilage, which is by now taking up the shape of the adult bone and is therefore known as the 'cartilaginous model', there is a steadily enlarging core of bone. At the same time the original cartilage is growing appositionally. A race develops between the two processes of cartilage deposition and bone formation, and continues until the adult stage of development is reached, at which time the bone formation 'catches up' with the deposition of cartilage so that the cartilage disappears, except for a thin rind which is left on the surface wherever the bone takes part in a joint with its neighbours.

Because the perichondrium has come to surround bone and not cartilage, we now call it periosteum, but it retains the same two layers. The perichondrium covering the cartilaginous joint surfaces disappears in the course of development. Such surfaces do not stop growing with the attainment of maturity, for they are exposed to considerable wear and tear which has to be made good, but reparative growth in this region is necessarily interstitial, as there can be no contribution from the perichondrium. Similar considerations apply to the articular cartilages at the ends of the long bones, which may retain a thickness of 5–6 mm in the larger joints.

Growth of long bones

The growth of the long bones of the limbs is more complicated. The primary centre appears in the cartilaginous shaft of the future bone in exactly the same way as in a short bone. But, about the same time, bone begins to be formed on the surface of the shaft, owing to the appearance of osteoblasts in the perichondrium, which now becomes the periosteum. The active cells in the deeper layer of the periosteum cause the shaft to grow in thickness. At the same time the bone formed in the primary centre is eroded away by osteo-clasts, leaving a cavity which is not built in by osteoblasts, and forms a convenient storage place for the blood-forming cells and fat which constitute the bone marrow. As ossification proceeds, so the marrow cavity extends along the shaft of the bone and at the same time grows in diameter because of osteoclastic activity in its walls. The bone continues to grow thicker by appositional growth on the outside of the shaft, but as it does so the destruction on the inner surface keeps pace, and in this way the ratio of the total diameter of the shaft to the thickness of its walls is maintained more or less constant until maturity.

While these events are taking place, the expanded ends of the cartilage model grow, at first by interstitial, and later by appositional growth. As time goes on, other centres of ossification appear in the cartilage masses at the ends of the future bone (Fig. 3.5). Such 'secondary centres' are, except for a few examples in reptiles and birds, confined to mammals; they are therefore not an essential part of bone growth in lower animals. In some sites two or three secondary centres may appear and eventually fuse together to form one large centre. A few secondary centres appear before birth, but the majority appear later, at a time characteristic of the individual bone; many do not begin their activity until puberty.

There is no relationship between the time of appearance of the various centres and the volume of bone they have to produce before growth stops; it follows that some of them progress much faster than others. The mass of bone formed by a secondary centre or an agglomeration of secondary centres is called an epiphysis, and, because of their calcium content, these epiphyses are readily seen in radiographs (Fig. 3.6), where they show as a dense shadow separated from the shaft by a translucent zone of still growing cartilage. This zone of cartilage is known as the 'epiphyseal plate', and is a vital factor in the growth in length of the bone.

Cartilage cells in the epiphyseal plate increase its thickness by interstitial growth at the same time as ossification proceeding outwards from the shaft is

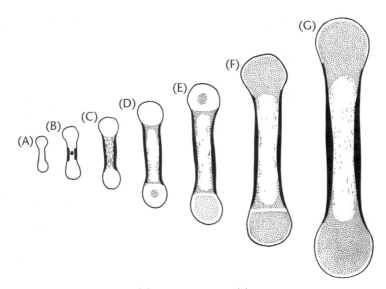

Fig. 3.5 Growth of long bone. (A) Cartilage model. (B) Primary centre appears in the shaft and a collar of compact periosteal bone surrounds it. (C) The shaft is ossified but the ends remain cartilaginous. (D) The marrow cavity appears in the shaft and progressively enlarges. A secondary centre eventually appears at one end of the bone. The walls of the shaft are made of compact bone. (E) Another secondary centre has appeared. The first has now formed an epiphysis of cancellous bone covered by cartilage and separated from the bony end of the shaft by a cartilaginous epiphyseal plate. (F) The second epiphyseal plate is overwhelmed by the ossification proceeding into it from the shaft and has been converted into bone. Growth at this plate has ceased and the epiphysis is said to be 'closed'. (G) The cartilaginous epiphyseal plate at the 'growing end' of the bone continues to grow in thickness for some time, but eventually it too is replaced by bone and growth in length comes to a halt. Throughout the whole process of growth in length, growth in thickness of the shaft has proceeded steadily by apposition from the periosteum.

destroying it and manufacturing bone. The result is that a race similar to that which occurs in the short bones takes place, and eventually the cartilaginous plate is overwhelmed, and becomes replaced by bone, which therefore unites the epiphyseal mass with the bony shaft. This 'closure' of the epiphysis terminates the growth in length of the bone, and in most of the long bones closure occurs at about the age of 16–18 years in the female and 18–21 years in the male. In rats some of the epiphyses of the long bones never close, but merely become inactive; such a quiescent zone of growth may be reactivated in fully adult animals. For example, rats can be made to grow at any time during their lives by injections of somatotrophin. This is not possible in humans once the epiphyses have closed.

One of the earliest things to be discovered about the growth of a limb bone was that interstitial growth in length does not occur. This was shown by Stephen Hales, and subsequently by John Hunter, who made marks on the shaft of a bone, allowed the animal to grow, and found that the distance between the marks remained constant.

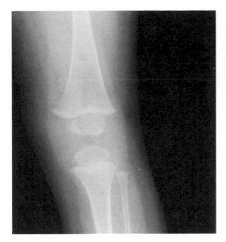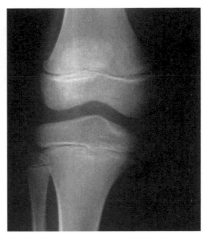

Fig. 3.6 Epiphyses. Compare the knee x-rays of an infant and those of an 11 year old. The lower end of the femur and upper end of the tibia in the infant both possess large rounded bony shadows, representing the secondary ossification centres. By the age of 11, these have developed into clear epiphyseal lines for the femur and also both the tibia and fibula. The patella appears as a white shadow over the femur and is also well ossified on this image.

Similar evidence has been obtained by embedding two pellets of metal in the substance of a growing bone and watching them grow. Both conventional radiology and magnetic resonance imaging are employed to study the growth of bone in association with other methods usually limited to animal investigations. For example, pigs readily eat the plant madder (*Rubia tinctoria*), which contains a compound similar to the dye alizarin. This is deposited where bone is being laid down and stains it pink. If an animal is given madder to eat for a known period, it can then be killed and the bones can be examined; all bone formed during the time of madder feeding will be stained pink, and will stand out from the normal white bone (Fig. 3.7).

There are a number of chemical compounds which can be used for their effects on growing bone. For example, the drug tetracycline is deposited mainly in the periosteal region, in the epiphyseal plate, and in the region at the end of the shaft and thus can be used to investigate the growth of these parts of the growing bone. Other techniques use radioisotopes to observe changes in growing bone employing the process of autoradiography.

In humans, more growth always takes place at one end of a long bone than at the other, and the more active end is sometimes known as the 'growing end' of the bone. This is perhaps misleading, as both ends grow, but the term does serve to indicate the end at which an injury might result in greater disturbance in the growth of the limb.

There are important differences in the behaviour of individual bones. Thus, the growing end of the femur puts on length roughly twice as fast as the growing end of the tibia. Injury to the epiphyseal plate at the lower end of

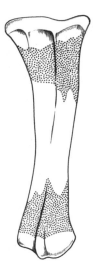

Fig. 3.7 Shaft of the tibia of a pig fed on madder. The madder was omitted from the food for 30 days before the animal was killed, and the bond formed during that time is white, while the previously formed bone is stained red (indicated by stippling). (Drawn from a photograph by Brash, J. C. (1934). *Edinburgh Medical Journal.* **41**, 305–19; 363–87.)

the femur is thus much more serious in its effect on growth than damage to the plate at the upper end of the tibia. If the growth at one end of a long bone is experimentally prevented, there is an increase in the rate of growth at the other end, but so far there is no explanation for this observation.

Just why one end of a bone should grow faster than the other is not known: the various influences which determine bone growth (Chapter 7) would be likely to affect both ends equally, and there appears to be no histological or biochemical difference between the epiphyseal plates of the two ends. It is similarly curious that in all long bones except the fibula the secondary centres which appear last are the first to fuse with the shaft. Occasionally, as in the rat, fusion does not take place at all, and the epiphyseal plate remains visible on a radiograph as a radiolucent line separating shaft from epiphysis. In such cases growth usually stops at or about the normal time. The pressure exerted by the growth process is enormous, and in order to stop growth at an epiphysis in a human limb it is necessary to apply a force of some 400 kg. Pressures less than this do not entirely stop growth, but they may impede it, and if the pressure is applied at an angle to the line of growth, deformities may result through the growth being misdirected. It has been suggested that certain deformities may be the result of faulty sitting or sleeping postures in small children; for example, the prone knee-chest sleeping position may give rise to bow legs through pressure being applied at an angle to the epiphyses at the knee.

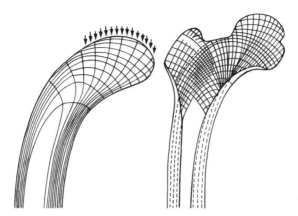

Fig. 3.8 Lines of stress in spongy bone. The upper end of the femur (right) compared with lines of stress in the head of a crane (left). (From Thompson, D'Arcy W. (1942). *Growth and form* (2nd edn). Cambridge University Press, London, by kind permission of the publishers.)

Growth is not uniform at different places within the same epiphyseal plate. This helps to maintain stability by producing ridging and grooving of the bony surfaces, and is also responsible for the 'cupping' of some epiphyses, such as the composite one at the upper end of the humerus, which fits over the conical end of the shaft of the bone.

At the ends of the bones, where growth is rapid, spongy bone tends to be produced. This has a honeycomb structure, in which thin plates of bone criss-cross each other, enclosing in their meshes little cellular spaces in which is packed the marrow. The directions taken by these trabeculae depend on the stresses thrown on the particular bone, for the collagen fibres, on which the inorganic salts are deposited, are laid down in such a way as to resist the pressure and tension lines of force in the bone. The most celebrated example is afforded by the head and neck of the femur, in which the stresses can be compared with the stresses in a crane head (Fig. 3.8). The trabeculae may at first be laid down at random, but those which are inclined obliquely to the shearing forces in the bone are moved out of the way by these forces. Trabeculae which happen to lie in the direction of a pressure or tension line will be comparatively undisturbed, as along these lines there is no shearing force. Nevertheless, a genetic factor is also involved, as bone removed from the body and grown in a nutrient medium will show similarly oriented trabeculae.

In the shaft of the bone, where growth is relatively slow, the bone produced by accretion is compact and dense. It has been suggested that rapid bone growth always produces spongy bone, and slow growth produces compact bone. Whatever the reason, the compact bone of the shafts of the long bones is thickest where it has to withstand the maximum stresses; in general, this is about the middle of the shaft.

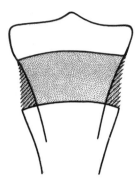

Fig. 3.9 External modelling of bone. The diagram shows the upper end of the tibia, the outline of the adult bone being superimposed on the outline of the 14-year-old stage of its development. The total amount of bone laid down by the epiphyseal plate during the time interval is shown by the stippling, and the amount of this bone which has to be removed in order to keep the contour of the tibia constant is shown by the cross-hatching.

Moulding and rearrangement is not confined to the interior of the growing bone. As growth proceeds, some of the existing surface material has to be removed if the characteristic shape of the bone is to be preserved (Fig. 3.9), and this is done by the osteoclasts. If anything goes wrong with the moulding process, the ends of the bones will be clumsy, thickened, and inadequately suited for their purpose. Some of the external moulding of a bone depends on the pressures and stresses exerted by the local soft tissues as, for example, the pull of muscles attached to the bone, or the pressure of a neighbouring nerve trunk. But these effects can only be considered as a kind of 'fine adjustment', and a bone grown in tissue culture, with no such influences acting on it, will still assume a shape not too different from the normal adult configuration.

Unlike the bone itself, the fibrous periosteum which covers it increases in surface area by general interstitial growth, and therefore some sliding has to take place between the two structures. As the muscles have their primary attachment to the periosteum, which is in turn attached to the bone by Sharpey's fibres, it follows that considerable local readjustments must occur in the case of muscles attached where much sliding takes place. The attachments of muscles have also to be rearranged because of the continuous moulding of the prominences or depressions to which they are fixed. Just as the distribution and arrangement of the trabeculae of spongy bone alter continuously to maintain the pattern induced by external stresses, the Haversian systems of compact bone which is undergoing moulding are removed and reorganized.

Once bone has been formed, it is by no means inactive; it is constantly being destroyed and reformed, and the picture presented by radio-isotope studies is one of an intensely busy tissue, in which the maximal rate of structural change occurs at about the age of $2\frac{1}{2}$ years. Destruction of trabecular bone tends to occur by removal of complete trabecular plates by osteoclasts rather than by progressive thinning and rarefaction. In young adults there is a relatively low turnover of material in bone, and the maximum bone mass in the skeleton has been achieved by the end of linear skeletal growth.

Later in life the amount of destruction gradually comes to predominate over the amount of replacement, so that bone tends to become rarefied and weakened in old age.

Growth of movable joints

The articular cartilage of synovial joints shows some response to stresses put upon it. For example, if a joint for any reason acquires an increased range of movement, the cartilage tends to extend in the required direction; this may occur even in adults. Conversely, if movement is restricted, part of the cartilage may become converted into fibrous tissue, and the articular surfaces may actually fuse together in places.

The thickness of the articular cartilage is proportional to the load in different parts of a joint; intermittent pressure stimulates growth, while continuous pressure inhibits it.

Body symmetry and asymmetry

One of the biggest challenges to our understanding of growth concerns the maintenance of symmetry between the left and right sides of the body as it is still unclear how the body ensures it grows to keep its two sides similar in size and how a cell knows the difference between left and right and up and down.

We all can recognize the minor degree of asymmetry that is always present in the human body. These asymmetries can be seen if you look for the small but often obvious differences in the face where there might be a slight difference between the shape of the right and left cheeks, mouth or the outline of the nose. The slight difference in size of the feet can make fitting shoes sometimes a problem. Such minor asymmetries are consistent right-left differences within the normal person and are usually of no major biological or medical significance.

More obvious asymmetry can occur in nature where a species has evolved to meet particular ecological situations. For example, fiddler crab males have an large right claw and the male narwhal has an elongated tooth on the left which develops into a tusk.

In biological and medical fields, asymmetry has been classified into three different classes, namely directional asymmetry, antisymmetry or fluctuating asymmetry. Each type has differing combinations of the right-minus-left differences.

Directional asymmetry arises when there is a greater development of part of the body on one side, for example, in the main body organs with the heart being located on the left side of the chest or where a leg might be longer on the right side than on the left side. These asymmetries only become important when they are associated with an abnormality of development or with disease. This type of body asymmetry is thought to be influenced by growth promoters during the development of the embryo such as the protein signalling molecules activin, lefty, nodal, and Sonic hedgehog (Shh).

Antisymmetry arises when the asymmetry is a normal part of the body character but is variable between one side or the other, for example human natural dominance where you may be right handed or left handed.

More difficult to understand as a concept is fluctuating asymmetry which occurs as a random deviation from perfect bilateral symmetry. This is related to developmental incidents when individuals are unable to undergo identical development of a bilateral character on both sides of the body. It occurs when small, random, deviations from a perfect bilateral symmetry in a body feature are present. An example of fluctuating asymmetry is the variation in human breast size that occurs during the menstrual cycle. In fact, fluctuating asymmetry is viewed as a measure of biological quality and may well provide important biological signalling mechanisms between individuals during growth and adulthood, playing a major part in sexual selection and reproduction. Unfortunately, scientific debate still has not resolved the most appropriate method of quantifying and analysing this form of asymmetry.

4 Growth of systems

I watched my foolish heart expand
Browning

Patterns of growth

Not all systems of the body follow the same pattern of growth. This is best illustrated by considering the development of the systems as a percentage of their attainment at maturity, taken at the arbitrary age of 20. Figure 4.1 illustrates the curve obtained for weight (solid line) plotted in this way. Similar curves are produced when the respiratory, digestive, and excretory systems are plotted on the chart, indicating that their relative sizes remain more or less constant during growth. The skeleton behaves in a similar manner, but some other important body systems follow different growth curves.

Lymphoid pattern

The lymph nodes and other lymphoid tissues such as the tonsils and thymus all grow rapidly in childhood and reach a maximum size by the age of puberty. A process of regression and degeneration then commences so that there is much less lymphoid tissue at the age of 20 than there was at puberty. Figure 4.1 illustrates the growth of the lymphoid structures, such as the tonsils, the thymus, and the lymph nodes.

Neural pattern

The central nervous system and the organs of special sense, together with the skull which contains them, follow a curve in which growth in the early stages of childhood is so rapid that the structures involved reach about 90% of their adult size by the age of 5 or 6 years (Fig. 4.1, dashed line). At 12 a child has a head which is almost as large as that of his father. From this time on, the growth of the nervous system is much slower than that of the rest of the body.

Gonadal pattern

A third pattern of growth is followed by the gonads and the external genitalia,

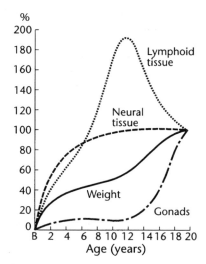

Fig. 4.1 The growth of systems and organs. Percentages of adult weight attained at plotted against age in years. (See text for description.) (Redrawn from Scammon, R. E. (1930). The measurement of the body in childhood. *The measurement of man* (ed. Harris, J. A., Jackson, C. M., Paterson, D. G., and Scammon, R. E.), University of Minnesota Press, Minneapolis, by kind permission of the publishers.)

which develop very slowly in the early stages, but at puberty begin to grow much faster than the rest of the body (Fig. 4.1, dashed and dotted line). Finally, the uterus and the adrenal glands share a fourth pattern, being relatively large at birth, actually losing weight rapidly, and not regaining their birth weights until just before puberty. Not only do the different systems and organs follow different patterns of growth, they also increase in absolute size and weight by very different amounts. Table 4.1 shows the approximate increase in weight from birth to maturity of a selection of organs and systems.

The skeleton

The total bone mass of the skeleton increases to a maximum in the third decade of life, and after this there is a slow diminution, as the osteoclasts begin to escape from control and the osteoblasts fail to replace the resorbed bone adequately.

The limbs

At birth, only the primary centres of ossification are present in the long bones of the upper limb, except for a centre in the head of the humerus. The upper limbs are also proportionately shorter at birth than in the adult, although they are long compared with the trunk and lower limbs.

Table 4.1 Weight increases from birth to maturity

Increase (approximate)	
30–40 times	Somatic muscles External genital organs Testicles Pancreas
25–30 times	Uterus
20–25 times	Body as a whole Skeleton Respiratory system
15–20 times	Heart Liver Lymphatic system Ovaries
10–15 times	Thyroid gland Kidneys
5–10 times	Pituitary gland
<5 times	Adrenal glands

In the lower limbs, primary centres of ossification are present in all the long bones, together with secondary centres in the head and lower end of the femur and the upper end of the tibia. The secondary centre in the lower end of the femur is used as a legal index of the full maturity of the infant. Compared with the upper limbs, the lower limbs are underdeveloped at birth and are held in a bent or flexed position.

Primary centres in the limb girdles are established early in intrauterine life, and by the time of birth have produced a considerable amount of bone (Fig. 4.2). In the pelvis, some secondary centres only appear at puberty and continue to grow until adulthood, often as late as the 25th year. These centres are often used in orthopaedic practice as a rough guide to skeletal maturity. In the foot, centres of ossification in the calcaneus and talus and the cuboid in about 50% of new-born, are present at birth. In the hand, the first bone to begin ossification is the capitate, the ossific centre, which appears some time during the first year after birth. Primary ossification in the long bones of the hand and foot (metacarpus, metatarsus, and phalanges) begins during fetal life so that the shafts are well ossified at birth.

The times of appearance of secondary centres in the limb bones are scattered over a long period, some being as late as the fourteenth or fifteenth year. The bone which they produce fuses with that produced by the primary centres at times varying from 16 years or so in the female elbow region to about 21 years for the male wrist region. The clavicle is usually the last long

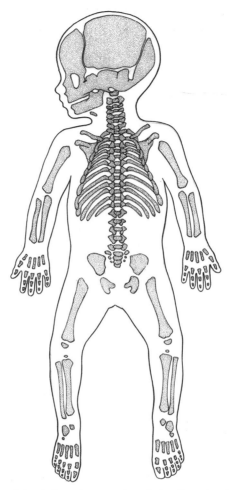

Fig. 4.2 Ossification of the skeleton in a new-born baby. Note the absence of any centres in the wrists, the separate centres for the components of the hip bones, and the lack of any secondary centres for the long bones except the lower end of the femur and the upper end of the tibia.

bone to stop growing, sometimes as late as the twenty-fifth year. The 'growing ends' of the long bones of the upper limb are the upper end of the humerus and the lower ends of the radius and ulna; in the lower limb the position is reversed, and the lower end of the femur and the upper end of the tibia undertake most of the growth in length.

The presence or absence of an epiphyseal line in a given situation at a given age is of considerable importance in the interpretation of radiographs taken after injury, for a perfectly normal line may be mistaken by the inexperienced for a fracture. Violence applied to a given region may result in displacement of an epiphysis if the patient is a child, while similar violence in an adult can only produce either a fracture or a dislocation of the adjacent joint.

At birth the bones of the pelvis and lower limbs are less advanced in relation to their ultimate size than those of the upper limb and shoulder girdle; they therefore have to 'catch up' by growing at a greater rate. Some of the most marked alterations in the skeleton occur in the pelvis. At birth the ilia and the sacrum are more upright than in the adult, and the subpubic angle is more acute, so that the cavity of the pelvis is not only very small, but also more funnel-shaped. After birth the growth of the pelvis keeps pace with the growth of the lower limbs. With the beginning of walking, the curvature of the sacrum increases, the ilia become thicker and stronger, and the acetabula become deeper. Later, at puberty, the characteristic sex differences in the pelvis become manifest.

The pelvic birth canal continues to grow for several years after the attainment of adult height, and the articular surfaces of the pubic bones show characteristic progressive modifications throughout life.

Skull and mandible

If the growth of the limb bones is complicated, that of the skull is more complicated still. At birth, the central nervous system is relatively very large, and consequently the vault of the skull, which contains the brain, also has to be large; its capacity is about 400 ml (adult 1300–1500 ml). After birth it follows the very rapid further growth of the brain; by the age of 2 years its capacity is approximately 950 ml, and its circumference has increased from about 33 cm to about 47 cm. The cranial vault is ossified in membrane, and at birth the bones which compose it are separated by gaps filled with fibrous connective tissue called sutures and fontanelles. These permit the bones to slide over each other to some extent as they pass through the narrow birth passages of the mother.

The largest gap is on the top of the skull between the frontal and parietal bones and is called the anterior fontanelle. It is about 3 cm across and is not filled in by ossification until the second year of life. It can become tense when the baby cries; sometimes, the pulsation of blood can also be observed through the membrane. Other fontanelles are shorter-lived (Fig. 4.3).

When the ossification process extends into the fibrous connective tissue, the individual bones of the vault come into relation with each other along a series of fibrous joints known as sutures. The edges of the bones are covered by a growing layer of osteoblasts and osteoclasts, and growth of the skull takes place at the sutures, at first very rapidly, and later more slowly. As the bones grow laterally, so additional bone is deposited on the outer surface of the vault, by the usual process of apposition from the periosteum. At the same

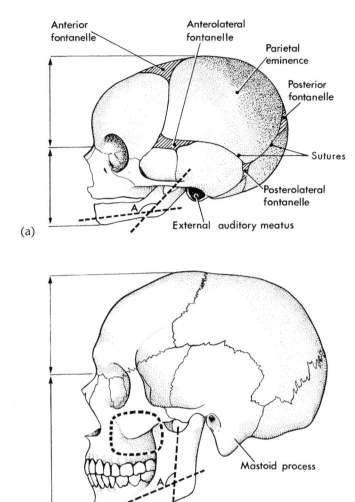

Fig. 4.3 Growth of the skull. (a) Skull at birth. Notice (i) the fontanelles; (ii) the smooth non-serrated suture lines; (iii) the absence of a mastoid process; (iv) the obliquity of the angle of the mandible; (v) the relatively small size of the face. (b) Skull of adult. Notice (i) absence of fontanelles; (ii) certain suture lines are now serrated; (iii) strong mastoid process; (iv) more upright mandible; (v) great increase in the vertical diameter of the face due to the eruption of teeth and the development of the jaws. The position of the maxillary sinus is indicated by the dotted line.

time, osteoclasts remove bone from the inside of the vault, so that the brain cavity grows in much the same way as the marrow cavity of a long bone (Fig. 4.4). As growth of the vault continues, remodelling processes convert the original single layer of bone into two layers of compact bone with a layer of

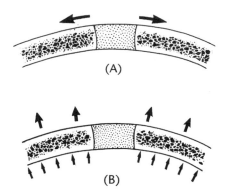

Fig. 4.4 Growth of vault of skull. (A) Growth at suture. The fibrous tissue separating the bones increases in amount and pushes the bones further apart. At the same time it is invaded by ossification spreading from the margins of the bones. (B) Appositional growth. New bone is added to the outer surface of the skull while excavation takes place inside, so maintaining the thickness of the vault relative to the total size of the skull and allowing the brain to expand concurrently.

spongy bone in between. The complexity of growth in such a system can be imagined.

After the first few years of life, many of the sutures of the vault come to interlock with each other like pieces in a jigsaw puzzle, and form jagged serrated lines; from this time on, growth at the sutures becomes a less important factor in increasing size, and it stops altogether about the time of puberty. Later still the sutures are obliterated, by extension of ossification into the sutural joints, and the individual bones become fused to each other. This obliteration may begin on the inner surface of the vault about the age of 25–30 years, and becomes visible on the outside of the skull some 10 years later, the sagittal suture usually fusing first. As with the obliteration of the epiphyseal lines in the long bones, there is great variation in the time at which the sutures close, but partial obliteration of the sagittal suture indicates an age in the early 30s, of the coronal suture an age of about 40, and of the lambdoidal suture an age of about 50. Occasionally, one or more sutures may close prematurely, and if this happens before much growth has occurred, deformities of the skull result which may require surgical treatment.

As growth proceeds, the contour of the cranial vault alters. For example, the parietal eminence (Fig. 4.3) which is well marked in the infant skull, becomes much less prominent in the skull of an adult, because surface apposition is more vigorous on the surrounding bone than on the eminence itself.

While the growth of the skull vault and orbit is related to the growth of the nervous system, that of the remainder of the face and the base of the skull is more closely associated with the growth of the muscles of mastication, including the tongue, and with the development of the teeth. The result is that the

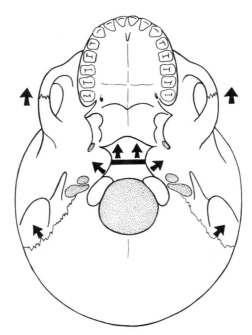

Fig. 4.5 Growth of base of skull. The main points at which growth in length and breadth take place are indicated by arrows.

base of the skull and face do not grow at the same rate as the vault and orbit. The base of the skull is formed in cartilage, and growth may continue here, at the joints between the ethmoid, the sphenoid, and the occipital bones (Fig. 4.5) until perhaps the twenty-fifth year, when the cartilaginous growing plate between the occipital and sphenoid bones is obliterated. This plate is the major site of growth in length of the skull. The face also grows for a similar time, the long period being related to the development of the jaws and the nasopharynx. It is for this reason that you do not acquire your permanent facial appearance until about the age of 25.

As the teeth develop, so the upper jaw is increased in size by surface apposition; bone is removed from its inner aspects to keep its proportions constant, and, concurrent with this, the bones of the face are excavated by osteoclastic activity to form the air sinuses which lighten the front of the skull. The largest of them is the maxillary sinus (Fig. 4.3), which grows in spurts following the times of eruption of the maxillary teeth related to it. The frontal sinus above the orbit excavates the frontal bone, which is at the same time added to by surface deposition to form the brow ridges. The increase in the length of the skull which occurs at the time of adolescence is largely due to this cause.

The mandible is very small at birth, and consists of two separate halves

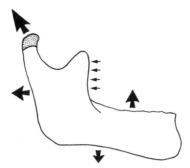

Fig. 4.6 Growth of mandible. Growth at the head of the mandible pushes the chin downwards and forwards. At the same time, appositional growth in the regions shown increases the vertical and horizontal dimension of the bone, while appositional growth on the outer surface increases its breadth. Absorption occurs on the front of the ramus, as shown by the small arrows, and on the inner surface of the bone to maintain the relative thickness constant.

joined by fibrous tissue in the mid-line. The two halves fuse during the first year of life, and the main subsequent growth of the mandible is in its length, although, as the mandible articulates with the skull, its width must increase to correspond with the width of the skull. The 'growing point' of the mandible at this stage is in the head of the bone, which lays down new bone by surface apposition, so pushing the mandible downwards and forwards. At the same time there is absorption of bone in front of the ramus and addition of bone behind it, so that more room is provided for the eruption of the teeth (Fig. 4.6). One consequence of this is that the angle of the mandible, where the ramus meets the body, becomes progressively reduced with increasing age from about 140° in the infant to about 120° in the adult (Fig. 4.3: indicated by (a)). This is part of the general increase in 'uprightness' of the face, much of which takes place at about adolescence.

The maximal growth activity in the region of the face at the time of the adolescent spurt is found in the mandible, which till then lags somewhat behind the rest of the face. Most of the growth at this time occurs in the ramus, but there is also a considerable increase in the length of the body and in the vertical height from the incisor teeth to the chin. Growth in the width of the face and jaws is completed relatively early; anteroposterior growth continues longer, and vertical growth longer still.

The vertical diameter of the orbit in the new-born skull is approximately equal to the distance between the lower margin of the orbit and the lower border of the body of the mandible (Fig. 4.3), and in the adult skull it is much less than this distance; the difference is due to the growth of the mandible and maxilla.

Teeth which have already erupted have to move forwards to make room for

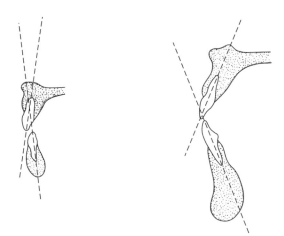

Fig. 4.7 Alteration with growth of the angle made by the incisor teeth of the upper and lower jaws.

the progressive eruption of the molars. The anterior walls of the tooth sockets are therefore continuously eroded, while bone is added correspondingly to their posterior margins. The deciduous incisors in the maxilla and mandible meet each other almost vertically, but their permanent successors slant forwards to meet at an obtuse angle (Fig. 4.7).

If the maxilla and mandible do not grow at the same rate, the eruption of the teeth may be interfered with, and various disabilities may follow the failure of the teeth to meet each other properly. The way in which the upper and lower teeth fit together (the 'occlusion') has a profound effect on the later stages of growth of the jaws.

The mastoid process does not begin to develop until after birth, and the associated bone forming the external auditory meatus is also deficient in the infant, and has to 'catch up' with the growth of the remainder of the bones on the side of the skull. It has been suggested that the growth of this region is stimulated by the pull of the sternomastoid muscle when the baby begins to raise up its head, but this is largely speculation, and the relatively minor influence of muscle pull on the shape of long bones lends it little support.

Vertebral column

The growth of various components of the vertebral column (spine) determine its overall adult length. These different components also have different growth rates which is reflected in their changes in proportion between birth and adulthood. The lumbar and sacral vertebrae are relatively smaller at birth in relation to their adult size when compared with the thoracic and cervical

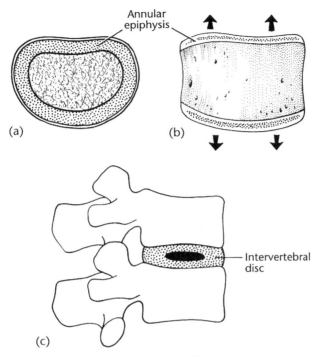

Fig. 4.8 Growth in height of vertebral column. (a) Body of vertebra seen from above, showing annular epiphysis. (b) Body of vertebra seen from in front, showing epiphyses. (c) Two lumbar vertebrae viewed from the side, showing the construction of the fibrocartilaginous disc between their bodies. The pulpy central portion of the disc is shown in black, surrounded by the fibrous part of the disc.

vertebrae and thus have to grow the most. The individual vertebrae grow in thickness by deposition of bone in the cartilage above and below the vertebral bodies and the appearance of the annular epiphyses in childhood allows the greater increase in length to occur at the time of the adolescent growth spurt (Fig. 4.8). These epiphyses do not close until well after most of the other bones of the body have ceased to grow. This can frequently be as late as the age of 25. The epiphyses in the upper thoracic region stay open longer than those elsewhere in the column.

Much less is known about the growth of the intervertebral discs, which account for one-quarter to one-third of the length of the vertebral column, and thus make a major contribution to the height of the individual. This contribution is variable, as the discs are compressible, and are therefore responsible for some of the diurnal variation in height. They are also highly dynamic structures, with changes in fluid content occurring rapidly over short periods between lying and standing. These observations have been made using magnetic resonance imaging and the changes could be highly significant to the causation of back pain in later life. Radiological investigation has shown that in children the disc below the eighth thoracic vertebra, after a period of growth around the time of birth, does not increase significantly in vertical diameter between the ages of 6 months and 8 years. On the other hand, the thickness of the disc below the fourth lumbar vertebra increases steadily up to the age of 2 years, and more rapidly thereafter.

Ribs and sternum

The sternum consists of the manubrium and a body made up of four segments which ossify from separate centres or pairs of centres. The bony body segments fuse together from below upwards, the first fusion being in early childhood and the last at about the age of 21.

The xiphoid process does not join the body until middle age, and the manubrium does not do so until old age, when the whole sternum becomes rigid, interfering with the movements of respiration. The ribs behave like long bones, and are well ossified at birth (Fig. 4.2). Secondary centres appear in the heads of all the ribs and in the tubercles of all but the last two pairs, fusing at about the twenty-fifth year.

Nervous system

In the new-born baby, the brain weighs about 350 g and accounts for 10–12% of the body weight. Males are slightly heavier than females. It doubles its birth weight in the first year of life and reaches 90% of its adult size by the fifth year when it has tripled its birth weight, but after this growth slows rapidly and progressively, so that it reaches 95% of its adult size by 10 years. The adult brain is only about 2% of the body weight. Although most of the major surface features of the cerebral hemispheres, called sulci and gyri, are present at birth, the cerebral cortex is only about half its adult thickness, and it is much more primitive in microscopic appearance. The spinal cord is about 15–18 cm long and extends so that its lower end is opposite either the second or the third lumbar vertebra. This is about one vertebra lower than in the adult so lumbar puncture is never attempted higher than the fourth lumbar vertebra in a new-born baby. In the adult, the spinal cord reaches a length of approximately 45 cm. This is because the spinal cord does not grow quite so much as the vertebral canal which contains it, and therefore appears to rise up in the canal.

At birth, the nerve fibres in the brain and spinal cord are far from completely mature, as many of those which will ultimately receive a coating of myelin have not yet done so. Myelination is not complete at birth; its most rapid phase of development occurs in the first 6 months of life, after which it continues at a far slower speed up to puberty and beyond, with myelination of the cerebral cortex continuing into adult life. At birth all the major sensory tracts are fairly well advanced, but the motor pathways are still undergoing a sequence of myelination. Not all the tracts and pathways in the nervous system are fully functional at birth and functional development runs independent of the progress of myelination. This leads to the new-born infant being able to undertake movements such as extension before flexion. However, the local reflexes related to swallowing and sucking appear before birth, and the fibres of the cranial nerves which subserve them have their sheaths. The optic pathways are well myelinated except for the optic nerves themselves, but the auditory pathways do not become myelinated completely until about 2 years of age.

Walking and locomotor control have traditionally been viewed as a series of stages, developing from simple reflexes through to complex neurological responses and inhibitions as the brain develops. However, today, it is generally accepted that upright walking in humans is a gradually emerging property which develops as the consequence of maturation of a number of body subsystems, including muscle strength and postural control centres in the brain.

In the skin there are marked changes in the neural pattern. During the third month of intrauterine life the epidermis begins to stratify, and it is immediately invaded by branches from the cutaneous plexus of nerves. But before birth, as the organized endings appear in the skin, the intra-epidermal fibres and endings withdraw, so that after birth only a few remain, although their number may increase in certain skin diseases. In the dermis of an infant, the organized sensory endings, such as the Meissner corpuscles, are closely packed together, but as the skin grows they become thinned out, much as spots painted on a balloon separate from each other as the balloon is inflated. There are therefore many fewer such end-organs per unit area in the adult than in the child. For different reasons there are fewer still in old people. It is not known whether a similar thinning out by separation occurs in the population of proprioceptive end-organs, such as muscle spindles, or whether the network of 'free' endings in the skin and elsewhere develops a wider mesh with growth.

The eye grows according to the neural pattern and reaches adult size by the age of 14. The eyeball is at first too short for its lens, so that most infants have about 1 dioptre of long-sightedness. As it grows, the eyeball becomes about 2 mm longer, but about 60% of the alteration in focusing that this enlargement would cause is eliminated by a concurrent reduction in converging power of the cornea and lens, so that the difference caused by growth just about cancels out the refractive error of the baby. The lens is peculiar in that it continues to grow throughout life, becoming about one-third bigger at the age of 60 than it is at 20. Secondary lens fibres are laid down in concentric layers around the existing primary fibres of the fetus. In this way, the primary fibres, plus the oldest secondary fibres, form the lens nucleus, and the younger secondary fibres form the cortex. The outer ear grows according to the general body pattern, but the inner ear, the middle ear cavity, and the eardrum are of almost adult size at birth and grow very little. In the infant the arachnoid granulations are small and few, but as the nervous system grows they become larger and more numerous, and bony excavations are formed in relation to them on the inside of the parietal bones alongside the superior sagittal sinus. These pits are radiologically prominent in old age, by which time the granulations may have reached a diameter of a few millimetres.

Cardiovascular system

The cardiovascular system undergoes a major change in its structure at birth due to the sudden imposition of major functional changes demanded by the achievement of independent living of the new-born baby. The fetus receives its oxygen from exchanges which take place between its circulating blood and that of the mother across the barrier within the placenta. There would be no point in driving its blood around the lungs, which are immature and only become capable of limited function from about 24 weeks of pregnancy.

Blood arrives in the fetus from the placenta by travelling along the umbilical vein. It then enters a special vein called the ductus venosus, which allows most of the blood to bypass the liver and pass to the inferior vena cava before it reaches the right atrium of the heart. Here, most of the richly oxygenated blood is largely shunted through a hole in the inter-atrial septum called the foramen ovale into the left atrium, so bypassing the pulmonary circulation (Fig. 4.9).

From the left ventricle it is circulated around the body, particularly to the head region, before returning to the heart by means of the two venae cavae. The deoxygenated blood from the upper part of the body, travelling in the superior vena cava, flows through the right atrium into the right ventricle in such a way as to avoid mixing with the placental blood from the inferior vena cava. Leaving the right ventricle, it flows into the pulmonary artery, whence the greater part of it rejoins the aorta through the ductus arteriosus, again bypassing the lungs.

As this inflow of venous blood to the arterial side of the circulation occurs farther from the heart than the origin of the main arteries to the head and neck and the upper limbs, these regions, especially the rapidly developing brain, obtain a better supply of oxygenated blood than do the abdomen and lower limbs. As already noted, the blood from the lower part of the body mixes with the arterial blood in the inferior vena cava, but there is only limited

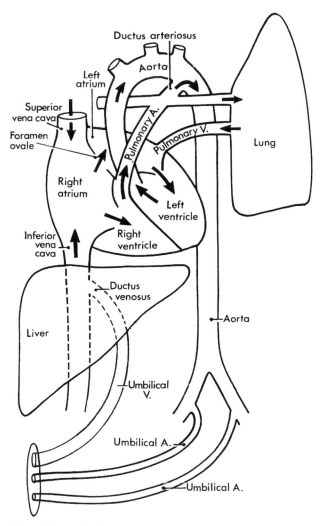

Fig. 4.9 Fetal circulation. The diagram omits everything except those features essential to an understanding of the main path of the blood—e.g. only one pulmonary vein is shown (see text for description).

mixing of the oxygenated and deoxygenated blood in the right atrium. The small and inactive lungs do not contain much blood in the earlier phases of development but a gradual, if small, increase occurs towards the end of gestation. Finally, the blood in the arterial tree is returned along the umbilical arteries to the placenta for reoxygenation.

At birth, blood flow from the placenta ceases, and the umbilical vein, the ductus venosus, and the umbilical arteries are very rapidly obliterated by muscular contraction of their walls initiated by the release of prostaglandins and accompanied by clotting of the blood within them. The vessels and their contents are eventually converted into fibrous cords by a process similar to the healing of a wound, and are then known, respectively, as the ligamentum teres, the ligamentum venosum, and the obliterated umbilical arteries.

The sudden shift of the site of oxygenation from the placenta to the lungs with the taking of the first breath means that the persistence of the pulmonary bypasses in the circulation would result in the blood not being properly oxygenated, and therefore the foramen ovale and the ductus arteriosus have to be closed.

The closure of the foramen ovale takes place in two stages. There is first a functional closure, which depends on pressure changes in the atria of the heart consequent on the flow of blood through the newly expanded lungs, and later an anatomical closure, in which the flaps of the valvular opening adhere together and fuse. Frequently, the anatomical phase of closure is incomplete, and a small hole persists between the two atria. However, so long as the hole is small and the pressure on either side of it remains more or less equal, there is little functional disturbance, although it may occasionally lead to problems in later life. On the other hand, should a substantial leakage occur from the right to the left side of the circulation, either between the atria or elsewhere, the blood circulated to the body may be incompletely oxygenated. In such cases there is often an interference with general growth.

The ductus arteriosus is also influenced to close by a sustained muscular contraction of its walls influenced by the release of prostaglandins. Like the umbilical vessels, it later becomes converted into a fibrous cord called the ligamentum arteriosum. If the processes involved in closure of the ductus fail to obliterate the channel, blood may pass from the aorta (high pressure) into the pulmonary artery (low pressure) and the resulting disability may require surgical treatment.

In the new-born baby the heart accounts for about 0.75% of the body weight, whereas in the adult the figure is only about 0.33%. This change is readily seen in radiographs, for in the infant the heart occupies some 40% of the lung fields, and in the adult only about 30%. The heart of the infant lies more or less transversely, and is later pushed downwards by the expanding lungs, so that in the adult it comes to lie more obliquely, and also lower in relation to the rib cage. The heart may continue to increase in size and weight during adult life, but much of the increase is due to the deposition of fat.

At birth, both ventricles have walls of similar thickness, but those of the right ventricle, in conformity with its less arduous task, grow less than those of the left ventricle, so that in the adult they are only about half as thick. There is quite a marked adolescent spurt in the heart muscle, and this is reflected in a rise in blood pressure, together with a slowing of the heart rate.

During normal growth there is little or no increase in the number of cardiac muscle fibres, but the cross-sectional area of each fibre increases by about seven times. As this happens, the number of small vessels increases, so that the number of muscle fibres supplied by each such vessel falls from about six in the new-born to approximately one in the adult. But because the whole system is increasing in size, the number of vessels per unit volume of tissue remains constant throughout. If the fibres in the heart wall are made to enlarge still further, there is no corresponding increase in the number of vessels.

Regarding the conducting system, there is a marked increase at birth in the amount of collagenous material among the fibres of the sinu-atrial node, and this is progressive with age. The nodal muscle fibres, unlike those of the atria, do not increase in diameter very much, and this may be because the atrial fibres have to perform against an increasing load, while the nodal fibres simply continue to initiate impulses and do not undergo mechanical stresses.

The arteries and veins grow in parallel with the growth in weight and height of the body; as they are called on to bear an increased pressure, so their walls thicken in response. Little is known about how blood vessels elongate to keep pace with body dimensions. Indeed, certain arteries grow longer than the distance which has to be travelled, and so become tortuous. In some cases the reason for this is apparent; for example the lingual artery is tortuous because it has to be able to stretch out to allow the tongue to be fully protruded. But in others, such as the splenic artery, it is not clear why the artery has to be tortuous or what stimulus to its growth brings it into this condition.

The number of valves in a given vein seems to remain constant during postnatal growth, and the evidence suggests that all the venous valves have appeared by the sixth month of fetal life. In experimental animals, arteriovenous anastomoses can be formed in response to increased local circulatory demand, and may disappear again when the stimulus is removed. Whether this occurs in humans is not known. Another response to the same stimulus is an increase in the density of the capillary network of the tissue concerned.

Haemopoietic system

At birth, red bone marrow occupies most of the spongy spaces and medullary cavities of the skeleton, but during childhood much of it is replaced by fat. By puberty none remains in the long bones except in the upper ends of the shafts of the femur and humerus; in the normal adult, red marrow is found only in the vertebrae and in the flat bones such as the sternum, the ribs, the innominate bones, and the scapulae.

There is a steady increase in the blood volume during childhood and also in the number of circulating erythrocytes per unit volume. The erythrocyte count is relatively high at birth, and falls together with the haemoglobin content of the blood, until about the third or fourth month after birth, when both figures begin to increase again.

During the adolescent spurt there is a considerable increase in both haemoglobin and the numbers of erythrocytes and at this time the erythrocyte count in boys rises above that for girls, and remains higher for the rest of life. At the same time, boys develop a considerable increase in the alkali reserve of the blood. These changes are physiologically necessary for the efficient use of the increased muscular development in the male, and the obvious conclusion is that they are mediated by some hormonal influence, but little is yet known about details.

The leucocyte count at birth is about 20 000 per mm^3, and falls to about 12 000 by the end of the first week, after which it gradually approaches the adult range; there is no adolescent spurt in the number of leucocytes.

Lymphatic system

Lymphoid tissue has a distinctive growth curve (Fig. 4.1), reaching its maximum development before puberty, and thereafter declining in both relative and absolute size, probably under the influence of the hormones produced by the gonads.

The thymus gland is a prominent feature of the chest of an infant, extending from the neck down into the anterior mediastinum and occupying much of the superior mediastinum. It weighs between 10 and 15 g at birth and this rapidly increases to about 20 g. It is intensely active, producing thymus-processed lymphocytes (T lymphocytes). These cells then mature and are exported via the bloodstream to the lymph nodes and other centres of lymphocytic activity throughout the body where they form self-supporting daughter colonies. They form a part of the human leucocyte antigen mechanism by which the body establishes its system of immunity. The thymus is at its largest size in the early part of life, reaching its maximum by about 15 years when it is at its peak of activity, after which it starts to undergo regression by the infiltration of fat into its structure. In the adult, it may be difficult to find as it appears to merge with the surrounding mediastinal fat. Although in the old person, it may be represented by a scanty mass of fibrous tissue, it usually has some active lymph tissue present.

After birth, the lymph nodes increase in size more than in number; the average total weight of the mesenteric nodes is said to increase nearly 20 times, but their number only about three times.

The tonsils and adenoids, so massive in the primary school child, usually settle down, unless they are diseased, to a very inconspicuous existence in the adult. Their maximum size is usually attained around the age of 6 years. The

Peyer's patches of the ileum also become much less obvious, and in old age may virtually disappear. The lymph nodes do not regress so dramatically, and may remain prominent, especially in the inguinal region, for many years of adult life. The spleen, which contains about a quarter of the total lymphoid tissue, grows with the general body growth curve rather than with the other lymphoid tissues, although its lymphoid component decreases along with the rest of the lymphoid system.

Respiratory system

The respiratory system is relatively very small at birth, but the lungs are not completely unexpanded, as some respiratory movements take place in the uterus. These partly fill the lungs with amniotic fluid, which is rapidly absorbed after birth. After the first breath, the lungs begin to grow rapidly; they increase threefold in weight and sixfold in volume during the first year. At the same time changes occur in the air passages. The terminal parts of the conducting tubes give rise to sprouts forming additional alveoli, and themselves become modified into respiratory bronchioles, while the existing respiratory bronchioles become modified into alveolar ducts. In this way the available respiratory surface area is increased, and at the same time the originally small conducting tubes rapidly grow in diameter. Altogether about six generations of conducting tubes are added to the bronchial tree after birth, most of the additions taking place in the first few months.

At birth there are some 20 million 'primitive saccules' (alveoli), and by the age of 8 years the number of alveoli has risen to about 300 million. In the later stages of growth the main feature is an enlargement of existing alveoli rather than further development of new ones.

Before birth the distal portions of the tree and the alveoli are lined by cuboidal epithelium, which flattens as soon as the lung is distended and respiration begins.

After the first few weeks the respiratory system follows the general growth curve, but, because the respiratory passages grow faster than the thoracic and cervical portions of the vertebral column, the larynx and trachea descend relative to it, so that the bifurcation of the trachea, which in the infant is opposite the third thoracic vertebra, comes to lie opposite the fourth by about the seventh or eighth year. The cricoid cartilage, opposite the fourth cervical vertebra in the infant has descended to the sixth cervical vertebra by the same time. The hyoid bone, which is level with the mandible before the onset of the adolescent spurt, drops rapidly at puberty to a somewhat lower level. The infant diaphragm, which is forced up by the pressure of the contents of the abdomen, descends to its adult position as the pelvis enlarges and the abdominal viscera descend.

The larynx enlarges slowly until puberty, when its growth speeds up in both sexes, but markedly more so in boys, the vocal folds doubling in length from 8 mm to 16 mm within a year; this is associated with the 'breaking' of the voice. Further growth subsequently takes place to the adult length of about 25 mm in the male and 20 mm in the female.

Digestive system

The development and eruption of two successive sets of teeth in a well-charted sequence affords a means of assessing the maturity of the child, and the process is considered in Chapter 5. The salivary glands triple their birth weight in the first 6 months, and by the age of 2 years are five times as large as at birth: at this stage they have acquired their adult structure. The tip of the tongue in an infant is usually stubby and rounded, and the mobile and more pointed tip of the adult tongue develops later, with chewing and with speech.

At birth, the tongue lies wholly in the mouth, but during the first 4 or 5 years of life its posterior part descends with the larynx and comes to form part of the front wall of the pharynx. The new-born baby is a nose breather and, until the tongue descends, the high position of the larynx and tongue allows him to continue to breathe freely while fluid is passing down on either side of the epiglottis and the uvula, which are in contact during swallowing. The oesophagus has a diameter of about 5 mm in the new-born, and both its upper and its lower ends are roughly two vertebrae higher than in the adult.

In the new-born baby the stomach is very small, having a capacity of approximately 30 ml, and lies horizontally. As feeding begins its capacity rapidly enlarges, tripling during the first 2 weeks. By the end of the first year it is capable of holding about 500 ml, and in the adult system its capacity often reaches 1500 ml. Like the respiratory system, the digestive system 'descends' with growth; the long axis of the stomach becomes more oblique, and the length of the small intestine is doubled by the time of puberty. The intestines at birth are very thin-walled because the musculature is not yet well developed; the mucosa and submucosa are more robust. Villi continue to form in the small intestine up to the time of puberty.

The posterior wall of the abdomen is relatively shallow in the infant; the lumbar curvature does not yet exist, and the vertebral column does not project so far forwards as it does in the adult.

Because the infant pelvis is small, very little of the small intestine can be accommodated in it; in the adult there is more room, and the small intestine, and indeed even the stomach, may extend into the pelvis. The caecum in the fetus is conical and the appendix is related to the apex of the cone. Differential growth later causes the caecum to descend relative to the abdominal wall, and greater growth of its lateral aspect alters its shape to a rounded cup; the appendix moves round to its inner side. The ileocaecal peritoneal recesses are usually more distinct in children than in adults.

The digestive organ which contributes most to the weight of the body is the liver, and at birth the liver is relatively large, its lower margin being palpable below the costal margin. At this stage it weighs 5% of the body weight, and this declines to about 2.5% in the adult. Its size at birth reflects the importance of the many functions which it is called upon to perform during intrauterine life.

Urinary system

The growth in size of the kidneys corresponds to the growth of the body as a whole. At birth the two kidneys weigh about 23 g; this weight doubles in 6 months and trebles by the end of the first year.

Like the brain, the kidneys are not fully functional at birth, and many of the renal tubules are not yet formed; the glomeruli enlarge considerably after birth, and in the new-born the cortex is much thinner relative to the medulla than it is in the adult. Probably no new glomeruli appear after the first few months of postnatal life. The kidneys of the new-born exhibit lobulation, which reflects their development in the embryo, but with growth this lobulation usually disappears, although traces of it are often still found in the adult. An important histological feature of the new-born kidney is the fact that the visceral layer of the capsule of the glomeruli is cubical rather than flattened. It is not until after the first year of life that this cubical epithelium is fully replaced by thin pavement epithelium, and during this year filtration by the kidney is relatively poor.

The growth of the kidney seems to depend on the physiological work it has to do; if one kidney is removed from an experimental animal, the remaining kidney can be induced, by a high-protein diet, to become larger than the two kidneys combined would have become.

The urinary bladder is an abdominal organ in infancy, but descends into the pelvis as the latter becomes more capacious (Fig. 4.10). The infant ureter is therefore relatively much shorter than in the adult, and has no pelvic portion In the infant the bladder is somewhat cigar-shaped, and it does not achieve its adult pyramidal shape until about the sixth year, by which time it has come to occupy more or less its adult position. In the infant the posterior surface of the bladder is completely covered by peritoneum.

Reproductive system

The gonads and external genitalia grow very slowly until the onset of the adolescent growth spurt (Fig. 4.1).

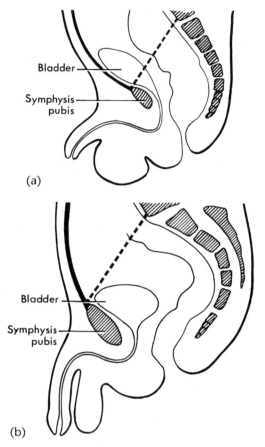

Bladder

Symphysis
pubis

(a)

Bladder

Symphysis
pubis

(b)

Fig. 4.10 Position of urinary bladder. Diagrammatic section through male pelvis. (a) Infant. The bladder is almost entirely an abdominal organ. (b) Adult. As the pelvis expands with growth, the bladder sinks into it, so that when empty it does not extend into the abdominal cavity.

During its development the testicle descends down the back wall of the abdomen and through the inguinal canal into the scrotum. By the time of birth it has usually arrived at its destination, or at least has descended beyond the superficial inguinal ring, but there are considerable variations in timing, and frequently the testicle does not descend fully until some years after birth. The processes involved in the descent of the testis are complex and probably require the presence of adequate levels of testosterone hormone during fetal development. As descent is necessary for the full maturation of the spermatozoa, a process which requires a temperature lower than that of the abdominal cavity, testicles retained in the abdomen, called anorchism, are probably infertile, with their seminiferous tubules becoming converted into fibrous tissue. Nevertheless, their endocrine function may be normal, and the secondary sexual characteristics may appear as usual.

The seminiferous tubules of a normal testicle are solid until puberty when they become canalized. During childhood, the testis remains small and grows slowly but at about age 10 or 11 it undergoes a marked acceleration of growth rate associated with the start of spermatogenesis and it acquires its characteristic resistant feel due to the pressure of the spermatozoa being formed inside it. The adult testicle is roughly 40 times as heavy as that of the new-born baby.

The prostate gland and the rectum are the only major organs in the male pelvis at birth. The prostate remains quiescent during childhood but at the time of the adolescent spurt, it enters a maturation phase when it suddenly doubles its size over a period of 6–12 months. It continues to grow more slowly for some years after puberty with the secretory component of the gland increasing relative to the musculofibrous tissue until after the age of 50 it may start to increase in size again.

At puberty, the seminal vesicles rapidly enlarge, and the mucous membrane lining them, which until this time has been thin and insignificant, becomes greatly thickened and folded. At birth, the penis is relatively large and the prepuce is often imperfectly separated from the glans; it may be some years before full separation takes place. The male urethra triples its length during postnatal growth, the spongy part growing most.

The ovaries at birth are small, although relatively large in comparison with the testicles. Like the bladder, they are abdominal organs in the fetus and infant, and enter the ovarian fossae by about the sixth year, just as the bladder is enabled to descend into the pelvis. Oogenesis is complete at or shortly after birth, and no new oocytes are formed afterwards. There is little growth of the ovaries until puberty, when the ovarian cycle begins, under the control of the anterior lobe of the pituitary gland. At this time the ovaries increase in size to a maximum of about 20 times the weight of the new-born organs. Before puberty the surface of the ovary is smooth, but after ovulation has become established it becomes progressively more and more scarred and 'cobbled'. During reproductive life the total number of oocytes becomes depleted from about 750 000 at birth to about 10 000 in women aged 45, although only some 450 ova are produced during that time.

The uterus is relatively large at birth, presumably owing to the influence of maternal hormones passing across the placenta. When this stimulus is removed, the uterus shrinks and does not regain its birth weight until the hormonal stimuli of impending puberty activate its growth again. The cervix of the uterus is considerably larger than the body of the organ until adolescence, when the body starts to grow so rapidly that it outstrips the cervix and comes to be double its length.

Because of the crowded situation in the pelvis, the uterus at birth lies in almost the same plane as the vagina. As the bladder descends into the pelvis, so the uterus bends forwards into its adult posture of anteversion and anteflexion when its position becomes variable depending on the contents of the bladder and rectum. The uterine tubes grow along with the uterus, in a similar pattern.

During menstruation, the organ becomes slightly enlarged and more blood vessels develop. In pregnancy the uterus grows dramatically, increasing its weight from about 50 g to nearly a kilogram at term. Most of the increase is due to growth of its muscular wall, in which the fibres increase in length, in thickness, and in number.

Changes in the blood supply and an increase in tissue fluid also contribute to the increase in size. The connective tissue components of the wall increase, and the endometrial cells enlarge and accumulate glycogen, becoming converted into decidua. The glands of the cervix form a thick mucous plug which blocks the cervical canal. As the pregnancy proceeds, the uterus expands upwards to appear above the symphysis of the pelvis by about 12 weeks and to reach the level of the umbilicus by 20 weeks.

There are two main factors responsible for these changes. The first is the growth stimulus provided by the hormones secreted by the corpus luteum of pregnancy and the placenta, and the second is the mechanical stretching of the uterine wall by its contents.

After delivery, the uterus contracts and begins the process of involution; by the end of the first week it weighs about 500 g, and by the eighth week it has returned to approximately its resting weight of approximately 50 g, although its cavity never returns to the pre-pregnancy size.

In both sexes the breasts may be enlarged in the period immediately after birth, and they often produce a certain amount of secretion as a result of stimulation by hormones such as maternal oestrogens and fetal prolactin. This is sometimes referred to as 'witch's milk', as it was a stigma made much of by some of the witch hunters in the seventeenth century. This activity rapidly subsides when the stimulus is removed. The breast then grows along with the general subcutaneous tissue until the time of puberty, when the female breast increases in size and becomes surrounded with secondary sexual fat (Fig. 4.11). New lobular structures are added to the developing and branching duct system, the nipple enlarges and the areola becomes more pronounced. Thereafter during each menstrual period, the breast usually slightly increases in size in mid-cycle due to increased blood flow and subsides again during and after menstruation. During pregnancy, more ducts and lobules are stimulated to grow within the breast by a complex hormonal mechanism and each breast gains about 400 g in weight. The culmination of this process occurs within 1–4 days of birth in the production of milk for the baby which can then continue for as long as 3 years if frequent suckling is maintained.

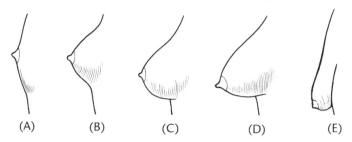

Fig. 4.11 Development of breast. Profiles of the female breast at different ages. (A) Childhood; (B) adolescence; (C) maturity; (D) pregnancy; (E) old age.

Endocrine system

The pituitary gland is relatively large at birth, weighing about 100 mg, and grows, like the thyroid gland, at a fairly steady rate (Fig. 4.12). However, the curve of growth is different in the two sexes, for the weight of the anterior lobe of the female pituitary is greater than that of the male; this superiority becomes evident fairly early in childhood, and is emphasized at the time of the adolescent spurt.

The parathyroid glands are relatively simple structures, with apparently only one type of secreting cell, until the age of 5 or 6 years when a second type of cell begins to appear; the functional significance of the change is so far unknown.

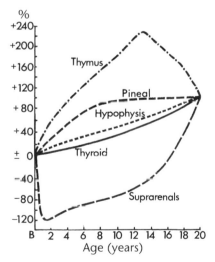

Fig. 4.12 Growth of certain internal organs. The curves show percentage of adult weight attained at a given time. From Scammon, R. E. (1930). The measurement of the body in childhood. *The measurement of man* (ed. Harris, J. A., Jackson, C. M., Peterson, D. G., and Scammon, R. E.). University of Minnesota Press, Minneapolis, by kind permission of the publishers.)

The thymus gland also has endocrine activity as well as its lymphoid role and as such is the largest gland in the body of the new-born relative to its body weight. It has an unusual growth pattern in that it increases in size up to puberty after which it undergoes a gradual reduction in endocrine activity. In the adult, it has a fatty structure containing endocrine tissue which continues to produce low levels of thymic hormones throughout life.

The adrenal glands have a growth curve similar to that of the uterus, but for a different reason. At birth, the glands are about a third the size of the adjacent kidney as they still have a thick cortex containing the characteristic fetal or transitional zone. By 3 months of life this begins to disappear and the three layers of the much thinner permanent cortex become established. As a result the glands become smaller, and only start to increase in size after 2 years so that they regain their birth weight by puberty (Fig. 4.12). In spite of a well-marked adolescent spurt, the adult adrenals increase little in weight, remaining about double the size of the new-born organs.

The prominent chromaffin tissues found in the paraganglia have reached their maximum size by about 8 months of pregnancy so that after birth they rapidly regress during growth. Thus the para-aortic bodies, which are maximal in size during the first 3 years and measure about 1cm in length, have completely dispersed by puberty, their function being taken over by the adrenal medulla which is not fully mature at birth.

Histological appearances indicate that the pineal body, like the thymus gland, is most active in late fetal life and early childhood. It synthesizes melatonin, a hormone implicated in the sleep-wake cycle, which is released at night and has a sleep-inducing effect. It may also be important in clearing free radicals from the body as a part of the ageing process. From the third decade onwards, adults accumulate calcareous deposits within cells of the gland, so-called pineal sand. As this is often detectable on a radiograph, it offers the radiologist a useful intracranial landmark especially if there is a tumour within the skull. About 10% of children over the age of 10 years have enough calcium in the gland for it to be detected by radiography.

5 Indices of maturity

... young boys and girls
Are level now with men
Shakespeare

Bone age

There are a number of important reasons why it might be necessary to assess the maturity of the child, especially in medical conditions which may affect growth and development. Clearly, the actual or chronological age of a child is a most unreliable guide to maturity as each child will mature at a different rate due to influences of its genetics, race, social background, and environment. The measurement of height and weight is also of very little value due to similar reasons. As a result, a number of methods have been developed which aid us in our estimation of the maturity of a child and allow us the opportunity to see if they are behind or ahead of their growth and development towards becoming an adult.

The most important of these methods is the assessment of 'bone age (also referred to as 'skeletal', 'anatomical', or 'radiological' age: the names are synonymous). During growth, every bone goes through a series of changes (Chapter 3) which can be recorded radiographically. The times of appearance of primary and secondary centres of ossification can be observed because the calcium content of the centres renders them radio-opaque, and the progressive enlargement of the ossified portion of an epiphysis or of a short bone can be followed in detail.

The sequence of the changes is roughly similar for a given bone in every person, but their timing may differ quite widely according as the local skeletal development is advanced, average, or delayed. As would be expected, there are exceptions to uniformity, and occasionally some of the centres may appear in an unusual sequence, but in general the course of events is reproducible enough to allow comparisons between different individuals.

Radiological examination therefore allows us to say how far the skeleton of a child has progressed towards skeletal maturity and thus adulthood. It would be unnecessarily dangerous to X-ray the whole body, and a sample of the general status of the skeleton is all that is generally taken. The wrist and hand

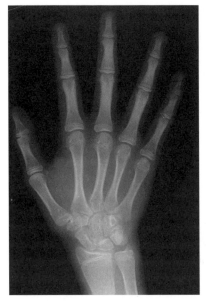
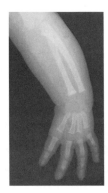
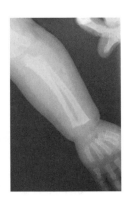

Fig. 5.1 Skeletal maturation. Radiograph of the hand of an adolescent compared with that of an infant of about 2 years of age. In the infant's hand, the secondary centre for the lower end of the radius appears as a wedge shape. The secondary centre for the ulna has not yet ossified. There are primary centres for only two of the carpal bones, the capitate (the largest) and the hamate. Secondary centres for the metacarpals and phalanges are present, appearing as small discs or circles adjacent to the end of the bones. In comparison, the adolescent's x-ray now demonstrates ossification of all the bones in the hand, although the final fusion of the epiphyses for the metacarpals, phalanges, radius and ulna has still not occurred.

are most commonly used for this purpose, as this region has a large number of centres of ossification. The risks of X-raying the hand are minimal, although the examination should not normally be undertaken unless there is a clear reason for doing it. Data on the hand have been available since the earliest days of radiology and its use as an index of skeletal maturation carries with it the assumption that the rest of the skeleton will behave similarly. Unfortunately, this assumption is not always true. Accordingly, in cases where there is a severe deviation from normal standards, other parts of the body may be used as a check.

At first it was thought sufficient merely to record the presence or absence of the centres in the hand and wrist (Fig. 5.1). But although satisfactory differentiation between stages of maturation could be achieved in the early part of childhood, in older children so few centres remained to appear that the procedure became less reliable.

Accordingly, measurements of the sizes of the centres were used. Eventually, it was realized that every centre of ossification passed through a number of morphological stages which have become known as 'maturity determinators'. These changes in the outlines of the centres are now listed in key diagrams.

Atlases showing skeletal development at different ages were constructed by Greulich and Pyle, and it is important to realize how these atlases took shape. First of all, large numbers of radiographs of children of a given chronological age were examined, and every individual bone was allotted a median maturity rating for that age.

An attempt was then made to find two single films (one male, one female) in which every bone would be as nearly as possible at the maturity rating already determined. These films were then accepted as the standard for that particular chronological age.

Such atlases have been of great use in child development studies and also play an important part in paediatric practice, particularly where hormonal problems are being investigated.

There are, however, three reasons why an atlas should not be relied upon too uncritically, quite apart from the fact that children of different socio-economic classes and different races mature at different rates.

The first is purely human, due to inherent unreliability of the atlases, as in use, estimates obtained do not advance smoothly, as in real life, but in a series of jumps.

The second is that there is considerable genetic variation in the order in which centres appear. The fact that a given centre has not appeared by its 'proper' time is therefore not necessarily an indication that skeletal maturation is delayed, and it is necessary to take into account the general appearances of every centre when coming to a decision. For example, the times for the hamate and capitate do not correlate well with those for the other centres.

The third objection is that arranging photographs in order of skeletal age implies a unit of measurement which may be called a 'skeletal year'. This unit, unlike a chronological year, is by no means constant; maturation does not proceed at a steady rate, and therefore to say that a child is a year behind the norm means very different things at different stages of development. Nor is it easy to fit a given radiograph exactly into position by extrapolating from one stage of development illustrated in the atlas to another.

For these reasons, the Tanner and Whitehouse scoring system (TW2) was developed, and nowadays it is common to rely on the 'percentage maturation'. Eight or nine stages are recognized for each bone, and points are awarded accordingly. The result is then reported as a percentage of complete overall maturation called the maturity score i.e. 100% score. A series of radiographs of children of different ages can then be scored and the results plotted on a centile chart similar to those used for height. The 'bone age' is then taken as the age on the chart at which the 50th centile score corresponds to the actual score of the child being investigated. The scoring system can use either the carpal bones (carpus) or the radius, ulna and the bones in the thumb and fingers (RUS) or use all 20 bones by including all the carpals and RUS bones which make up the component scoring systems. In clinical practice, while it is often found satisfactory only to score the radius, the ulna, and the finger bones, the total 20 bone score provides a more accurate overall score.

The TW2 method uses only one set of standards for both males and females: the female scores are simply higher than the male ones. The Greulich and Pyle atlases were compiled from well-off American children, whereas the TW2 scoring system was derived from a randomly selected group of Scottish children, who were about 6 months less advanced. The two methods therefore give different standards, and a correction is necessary if they are to be compared.

The reason for using such methods is to be able to say whether a child who comes for examination is skeletally retarded, 'normal', or advanced, and the next difficulty is immediately obvious. What criterion distinguishes the 'normal' from the 'abnormal'? Is a difference of 2 years on the atlas sufficient? Should the difference be so many points on the scoring system? This is exactly the same difficulty as faced us when dealing with the growth charts for height and weight, and there is no hard and fast answer. Individual variation in maturation of the skeleton, like individual variation in growth, is so considerable that it is quite possible for a child at one stage of development to be widely separated from the median maturity picture without this necessarily implying any deleterious effect on his or her future. However, if serial checks at intervals of 6 months or a year show a consistent or increasing deviation from the median, the matter has to be regarded more seriously. Even so, radiological age is only one factor in a general examination of the patient. If there is any suspicion that the hand may not be reflecting a true indication of general progress, radiographs of other regions may be taken, and a composite report obtained. For example, a case is cited of an undernourished 8-year-old child whose overall skeletal age was thought to be just over 5 years, but who had some bones at $2\frac{1}{2}$ years development, and others at $6\frac{1}{2}$ years development.

Several different methods have been developed for assessment of the maturity of the knee and there are also standards available for foot and ankle. In the first year of life they give a better indication of bone age than the hand.

Skeletal maturation usually proceeds roughly parallel with skeletal growth, and, of course, maturation and growth both come to an end when the epiphyses close. The factors influencing skeletal maturation are similar to those which control growth, and will be discussed in Chapter 7. Prominent among them is sex, for at every chronological age up to full maturity the radiological age of girls is in advance of that of boys by about 20% or more.

Dental age

Another series of convenient landmarks by which the development of the child may be estimated is provided by the times of appearance of the primary and secondary dentitions. The primary teeth begin to calcify during the fourth to sixth months of fetal life, and at birth some of them are more advanced than others. At about 6 months of age, the mandibular incisors (usually) are the first of the primary teeth to erupt; that is, to appear wholly through the gum. At this stage calcification of the primary teeth is not yet complete, and it does not become so until about 3 years of age. The crowns of some of the permanent molars are by this time fully developed, and their roots are beginning to form. At 6 years of age the mouth is said to be 'full of teeth', as at this time there are more teeth in the jaw than at any other. The teeth of the primary dentition have not yet begun to fall out, and those of the secondary dentition are more or less fully formed. Shortly after this, the primary incisors are shed, and the first permanent molar erupts. A series of complicated changes takes place in the jaws to allow room for the larger secondary teeth to occupy the limited amount of space left by the shedding of the primary teeth, and it is at this time that many of the difficulties caused by crowding of teeth may become apparent.

The radiographic appearances of the developing jaws and teeth give the most accurate information. Maturity staging by this means takes into account such factors as calcification and the completion of crown, cusps, roots, etc. in addition to eruption of the teeth. However, most estimates are based simply on the times of eruption of given teeth, and the simplest method of obtaining the dental age requires nothing more difficult than enumerating the secondary teeth present; recourse to a table gives the dental age. The mean times of eruption of the secondary teeth are shown in Fig. 5.2, but this sequence is far from invariable, and the diagram gives little indication of the probable course of events in any single person. Nevertheless certain teeth appear at fairly predictable times.

One of these is the second permanent molar, which erupts at about 12 years of age. Because of its regularity it was once used in Britain as an indication of whether a child was old enough to go to work in a factory under the terms of the Factory Act, and accordingly it was named the 'factory tooth'. In an era when documentation of chronological age was far from complete such a test had its value.

The third permanent molar erupts at any time between the ages of 18 and 80, and is useless as a marker; it was called the wisdom tooth on the assumption that it appeared about the age of discretion.

There is no sex difference in the eruption of the primary teeth, but, just as

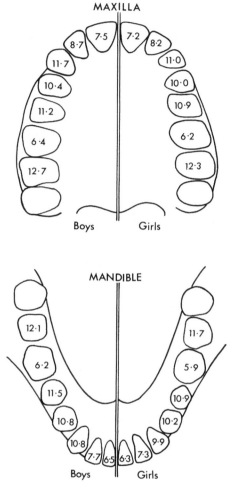

Fig. 5.2 Mean times of eruption of the permanent teeth. Note that the first to appear is usually the first permanent molar in the lower jaw. The times of appearance of the third molar ('wisdom') teeth are so variable that they have been omitted.

girls are ahead of boys in skeletal maturity so they lead in the secondary dentition, the biggest difference being in the times of eruption of the canines (Fig. 5.2).

Difficulties in assessment are introduced by the fact that some investigators have taken 'eruption' to mean the time of first appearance of any part of the crown of the tooth through the gum, while others have waited until the whole of the crown has pushed its way through; there is often a considerable interval between the two stages. Eruption is in fact only one event in the ossification process and has no real biological meaning. For this reason, Demirjian in Canada developed a useful series of scales which can be applied to the assessment of dental maturity using principles developed by Tanner in his TW2 Atlas.

Nevertheless, dental age can supplement bone age in the estimation of maturity, both in paediatrics and in criminology. Just as the condition of the skull sutures can be used to obtain a very rough estimate of the age of an adult, so can the condition of the tooth enamel. This, the hardest material in the body, is gradually worn down by a lifetime of eating, and the amount of wear is permanent, as the enamel organ of the tooth dies when it has completed its work, and enamel cannot be renewed. Wear depends not only on age, but on the type of food eaten, and anything like accuracy is impossible. Unlike such creatures as the shark, humans do not have a reserve dentition, and if a tooth of the secondary dentition is lost, there is no replacement. Such losses are not due to age, but to disease affecting the gums and teeth themselves.

Sexual age and puberty

As the child grows up, the development and maturation of the sexual organs mark the onset of puberty and these changes have been used to supplement the meagre information afforded at this time by radiographic and dental studies.

Legally, puberty is the time at which the individual becomes functionally capable of producing a child; in England this state is recognized by the law courts to have been reached by the ages of 12 for girls and 14 for boys.

Medically, the word 'puberty' is applied to a series of events spread over several years, with a sequence and timing which vary from person to person. It is the transitional stage from childhood to adulthood. However, the process of sexual maturation takes place over the growing period of the child, starting during fetal development and ending on attainment of full maturity. In the fetus, the gonads undergo differentiation into female and male while maturation occurs during the postnatal development which culminates in puberty. The events marking puberty commence well before any physical signs of puberty are present and are driven by pulsed release of gonadotrophic-releasing hormones from the hypothalamus in the brain. The presence of these hormones can be detected as early as 7–8 years of age in girls and about a year later in boys.

The rate of progress of the changes of puberty is independent of the time at which it begins, with its duration varying from about 2 to $4\frac{1}{2}$ years. About 50%

of children complete the sequence in 3 years, and virtually all do so in 5 years. Children who begin to develop early are thus not necessarily the first to reach sexual maturity.

The process of puberty is driven by the release of hormones from the hypothalamic-pituitary-gonadal system. The pulsed release of the hypothalamic gonadotrophic-releasing hormone occurs initially during the night but gradually then takes place throughout the 24 hour period. A marked influence on the whole process of puberty has been attributed to the nutritional status of the individual. This has led to the hypothesis that early childhood environmental influences on puberty may in turn have an effect on fertility in later life (see Chapter 8).

The earliest sign of male puberty is the growth of the testicles. This may occur as early as 9 years or as late as 15 years, and may be measured with an orchidometer, which is simply a series of plastic ovoids of known volume strung together. The ovoid most closely corresponding to the size of the testicle as determined by palpation is taken as giving the volume of the organ. The average adult testicle has a volume of about 20 ml, and a volume of 6 ml may be taken as indicating that puberty has started. At this time mitotic figures abound in the seminiferous tubules, spermatogenesis begins, and testosterone appears in the urine. The penis, prostate, and seminal vesicles begin to enlarge, and this is followed by changes in the larynx, the skin, and the distribution of the hair on the body. The timing of the growth spurt of the penis is subject to just as wide variations as the timing for the spurt in height, and at the age of 14 some boys may be practically mature sexually, while others have not even begun their sexual spurt. It is useful clinically to remember that whatever his age, a boy in the early stages of sexual development has usually not begun his maximal rate of growth, and will subsequently add considerably to his height.

The acceleration of the growth of the larynx does not occur until about the termination of the penile spurt, and is presumably due to a direct stimulation of the cells of the laryngeal cartilages and the associated soft parts by testosterone.

Pubic hair may appear before the spurt in height has begun, although it is usually somewhat later. There are racial differences. Other body hair, such as axillary and facial hair, usually does not appear until about 2 years or so after the first appearance of the pubic hair. The scrotal skin also darkens. The first ejaculation of semen usually occurs within a year of the beginning of the enlargement of the penis (Table 5.1). The apocrine sweat glands of the axilla and genital regions also are thought to increase in number at puberty, and certainly are aroused to activity at this time.

Boys may also have some enlargement of their breasts accompanied by an increase in the diameter of the areolae.

Table 5.1 Rough timetable of sexual maturation

	Boys	Girls
Onset	Testicular enlargement begins Seminiferous tubules canalize Primary spermatocytes appear Fine downy straight pubic hair appears	Ovarian enlargement begins Breasts develop to 'bud' stage Fine downy straight pubic hair appears
A year or more later	Secondary spermatocytes present Penile enlargement progressing Pubic hair now coarser and curling	Pigmentation of areolae Pubic hair now coarser and curling
A year or more later	Relative enlargement of larynx beginning First ejaculation	Relative increase of pelvic diameter beginning Menarche; first cycles may not produce ova
A year or more later	Mature spermatozoa present Axillary hair Sweat and sebaceous glands very active	Full reproductivity Axillary hair Sweat and sebaceous glands very active

Box 5.1

In clinically assessing puberty and its development, the paediatrician needs to be able to recognize different stages of puberty accurately. Tanner devised a clinical scoring system based on five stages of a boy's pubic hair development. These are:

(1) no different from hair on the rest of the abdomen;

(2) slightly pigmented, longer, straight, and often still downy;

(3) definitely pigmented, and curly round the base of the penis;

(4) adult in type but not in extent: boundary at inguinal fold;

(5) spread to medial surface of thigh;

(6) spread along linea alba.

In the female, the ovaries, like the testicles in the male, increase in size as the first sign of puberty, but this cannot be detected except at operation, although the quantity of oestrogens excreted in the urine gives an indication of ovarian activity. The first external sign of female puberty is the enlargement of the breasts, which precedes the maximal velocity of the adolescent spurt, and begins on average between 9 and 13 years of age. Internally, in the female reproductive tract, changes in the vaginal epithelium are occurring. It thickens and accumulates glycogen. The bacterial flora in the vagina change and the reaction of vaginal fluids changes to one of acidity.

Box 5.2

In the female, puberty ratings can be assessed using stages of breast and pubic hair development.

There are five stages of breast development:

(1) only the nipple is raised above the level of the breast;

(2) bud-shaped elevation of the areola, which increases in diameter;

(3) elevation of the breast and increase in diameter of areola;

(4) increasing amounts of fat deposited; areola often elevated;

(5) areola subsides to level of breast

It should be noted that about the time the breasts begin to enlarge, the growth of the uterus and vagina accelerates.

Six stages of the development of the pubic hair can be defined:

(1) no specialized hair in the pubic region;

(2) scarcely pigmented hair, especially along the labia;

(3) sparse dark curly hair on labia;

(4) hair adult in type but not in extent;

(5) lateral spreading;

(6) further extension upwards and outwards.

Age of menarche

Several stages in sexual development have been recognized for the purpose of estimating the sexual age. The maturation of the female breast has been subdivided into five stages (see Box 5.2), and so has the maturation of the female pubic hair. But by far the greatest amount of work has been done in relation to the onset of menstruation (the menarche), which occurs anything up to 4 years after the first sign of breast development, the average interval being about $2\frac{1}{2}$ years. A continued decrease in the age of menarche has been recognized in Europe from the mid-nineteenth century onwards. This rate was about 4 months per decade, with variations between countries. It is now reported that this decline has stopped in some countries. The reasons for this effect are attributed among other things to nutritional factors and there is a relationship with social class. This points clearly to the important role that the environment external to the body plays in growth and maturity.

The age at which the periods first start is an event which is well remembered by the subject, and theoretically can be timed with accuracy, although there are difficulties in collecting data. For example, if women are questioned retrospectively their recollection may differ according to their age at questioning, and dates tend to be clustered around birthdays, school terms, and so on. A second method is much more accurate, but involves smaller numbers, as it consists in following a group of children longitudinally until the menarche occurs. A third method depends on analysing the percentages of children of accurately known ages who have already started menstruating.

The menarche does not occur until after the peak of the spurt in height is over (Fig. 5.3), and corresponds to the period of maximal deceleration of growth. A girl who has begun to menstruate can be told with confidence that

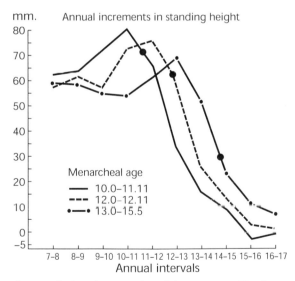

Fig. 5.3 Time of menarche in relation to the adolescent spurt. The three velocity curves for height represent the growth of early, average, and late maturing girls, and the black circles show the average time of menarche for each group. Notice that the menarche occurs after the peak velocities have begun to decline. (Slightly modified from Simmons, K. and Greulich, W. W. (1943). *Journal of Pediatrics*, **22**, 518–48, by kind permission of Professor Greulich and the editor.)

her growth is rapidly slowing down, and that she is unlikely to grow more than another 8 cm at most. Many of the early menstrual cycles may not involve ovulation, and full sexual maturity may therefore be delayed for a year or two after menstruation has begun. Conversely, cyclic liberation of ova may occur in some girls earlier than the onset of menstruation.

Fertility is low at the time of menarche but rapidly rises to a high level during the early adult years before falling off as the age of cessation of periods (the menopause) occurs. This has important biological and medical implications as it might be a way of protecting very young mothers from becoming pregnant before the body is prepared for it. There is a considerable body of medical evidence which indicates that the young mother carries a high risk of problems in her pregnancy with her baby more likely to be premature and under-weight. Other factors which may lead to problems include the immaturity of the maternal pelvis and the continuing growth of the body. Before adult maturity and the cessation of growth, the body still has not achieved optimal nutrition and this can also affect fetal development. As described elsewhere, this indicates that child bearing ideally should not commence until into the mid-twenties.

The age at which the menarche occurs is more closely related to the radiological than to the chronological age. Thus, menstruation nowadays begins within a chronological age range of 10–16 years, but within a much narrower range of radiological age from 12 to $14\frac{1}{2}$ years, at about the time of fusion of the epiphyses of the terminal phalanges of the fingers.

Tall girls reach sexual maturity earlier than short ones, but girls with a late adolescent spurt and late puberty are ultimately taller on the average than those who begin menstruating earlier, for they have longer in which to grow. The birth order also has some effect, as puberty occurs earlier if there are several older brothers and sisters; the difference between the firstborn and the sixth child may be as much as a year. It has been suggested that the menarche occurs when the critical weight of about 47 kg is reached; different races may have different critical weights. In animals, weight is more important than chronological age in determining the onset of puberty, and it is possible that the attainment of a critical weight might involve a change in metabolic rate which could trigger off the hormonal changes necessary for puberty. Certainly malnutrition, either involuntary or voluntary, as in anorexia nervosa, delays the menarche. Female athletes and ballet dancers may have a delayed menarche, perhaps because rigorous training and slimming cause a weight loss of 10–15% of normal weight for height; this is regarded as the level at which menarche is delayed, or, in an adult, menstruation is abolished. Other factors, however, are also operative. Thus, twins have a later menarche than singletons, and emotional stress will delay the menarche or abolish menstruation if it is already established.

Despite the plausibility of the critical weight for height theory, recent evidence derived from the study of over 4000 girls at the age of 11 years has shown that relative weight explains only a small proportion of the variation in age at menarche. It is probable that in normal girls most of the variation is in fact genetic.

Enlargement of the testicles before the age of 9 or of the female breasts before the age of 8, followed by the normal development of other signs of puberty, is classified as 'central' precocious puberty (due to the activity of the hypothalamic-pituitary-gonadal axis; see Chapter 7). It is four to five times more common in girls, and must be contrasted with the distorted precocious puberty due to overactivity of the adrenal glands.

On the other hand, delayed puberty is a common cause of worry to the individual and to his or her family. There are many possible causes, but most are relatively uncommon, and the usual type, particularly in boys, is 'constitutional delayed puberty', which is probably genetic in nature. Over 95% of boys and girls show some signs of puberty by the age of 16, and delay beyond this time merits investigation.

All the events of normal puberty appear to depend on the action of the pituitary hormone gonadotrophin, and this can be used in the treatment of delayed puberty. It is important that treatment is initiated early, so as to avoid anxiety and distress.

Estimation of chronological age from anatomical data

The determination of chronological age is required for legal purposes when dead bodies have to be identified or when an attempt has to be made to establish whether or not a person has reached the age at which the law recognizes responsibility. More often the problem concerns the age and identification of the victim rather than that of the murderer. A celebrated historical example is that of the 'Princes in the Tower', whose skeletons were subjected to anatomical investigations in order to try to pin-point the date at which they were done to death, and so to establish whether Richard III or Henry VII was responsible.

The wide range of biological variation makes it impossible to say exactly how old a person is. A probability can be established by anatomical examination, but nothing more. In adolescence one can only be accurate to within 3 or 4 years, and in later life the margin is much wider, as after the epiphyses have closed there is less to go upon and imprecise indications such as the fusion of the skull sutures, the calcification of the rib cartilages, the obliteration of the sternomanubrial joint, or the appearance of the pubic articular surfaces have to be used. It is also possible to correlate the known age of long bones with information obtained by scanning their radiographs with a microdensitometer.

Neural age

In spite of the large size of the central nervous system at birth, much of it, as has already been pointed out, is incompletely functional and requires a considerable time to develop to the stage at which it can be utilized to the full. A new-born baby has a limited repertoire of purposeful activity, being able to cry, suck, swallow, sneeze, move the eyes, defecate, and micturate. Although there is a sense of taste and smell, it is uncertain how far the sense of pain has developed as there are views that pain can be felt by the developing fetus. There is also a remarkably powerful grasp reflex, which is lost within a couple of months of birth.

The human baby faces two main difficulties which are not shared by most other animals. There is a considerable reliance on learning rather than inherited behaviour, and the skills necessary to hold the body upright against the force of gravity must be developed. Furthermore, the baby has to learn to use the upper limbs as tools with which to manipulate the environment. It is not surprising, therefore, that motor and sensory development are slow, and that progress can readily be followed in the growing child, and made use of as an index of maturation. A good example is the way in which the random swings of the upper limbs in the baby gradually become refined into purposive handling behaviour; the parts of the limbs nearest the trunk come under control before the more distant parts. A great deal of detailed work has been done on this type of development by Gesell and his colleagues in America, and by others in Britain: it is impossible to give a proper account of it in a book of this size, but certain landmarks of development are shown in Table 5.2 and in Fig. 5.4, which give an idea of the scope of such investigations.

Girls are ahead of boys throughout the phase of motor and sensory development: they are first to acquire the movements necessary for crawling and walking, and first in the development of skills which need fine movements and co-ordination, such as tying bows. They learn to control their bladders earlier than boys. One of the landmarks commonly recorded by mothers is the age at which their babies say their first word. This occurs at a very variable time, but by about $1\frac{1}{2}$ years of age approximately 30 words are accurately used. By 2 years this number has risen to about 300, girls being more advanced than boys. By the age of 3, the child probably knows more than 1000 words, and by 5 more than 2000. The combination of words into language has progressed far enough by the age of 3 for nearly all children to use at least three words per sentence; a child of 5 years can usually use more than five words per sentence, but there

Table 5.2 Developmental landmarks

Years	Age Months	
—	2	Follows moving objects with eyes
—	4	Can sit propped up for a short time; moves head to inspect surroundings
—	6	Grasps objects; begins to bang and shake them
—	8	May sit unaided
—	10	Creeps; picks up small objects between finger and thumb; one or two words; tries to help with feeding
1	—	'Cruises' holding on to rail of cot; Walks with one hand held; throws objects on floor; co-operates in dressing; waves goodbye; puts toys in and out of container
1	6	Walks; runs awkwardly and stiffly; builds towers of 3–4 blocks; can turn pages of a book; about 30 words
2	—	Runs without falling; uses three-word sentences; can turn door knob; obeys simple instructions; builds towers of 6–7 blocks; bowel and bladder control sometimes good
3	—	Walks erect; can stand on one foot; climbs; can put on shoes and unbutton some buttons; bowel and bladder control usually established; eats reasonably well by himself; counting begins
4	—	Draws, copies, prints letters; cleans teeth, washes and dries face and hands
5	—	Can lace shoes and is beginning to use tools; some are reading quite well and most can write their own names; questions about meaning of words
6	—	Reads; balls are bounced and (sometimes) caught

N.B. The information in this table is only approximate and does not fit every child.

are very great variations in this, as in other phases of psychological development.

The maturation of psychological awareness involves progression from completely self-centred absorption to the recognition of the existence of others and finally to the development of an adult appreciation of the individual's

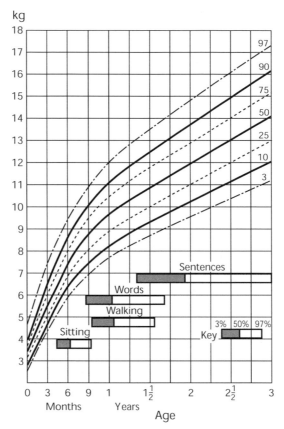

kg

Fig. 5.4 Developmental landmarks and growth in weight (centile standards) during the first 3 years of life (English girls). (From *British Medical Journal* (1971), **2**, 125, by permission of the editor, Professor S. D. M. Court, and Dr. G. A. Neligan.)

place in society. In learning to cope with problems, boys are more aggressive than girls, who tend to ask for help more quickly, or to collapse in tears. On the other hand, boys have a shorter attention span. Additional evidence on the development of personality is afforded by the artistic productions of the child, which give an indication of the progress of ideas and skills; it is often possible to differentiate sharply between male and female efforts of this kind.

Mental age

There have been many attempts to devise performance tests which measure the elusive quantity conveniently described as 'intelligence', and some of these, such as the Stanford-Binet Test and the Wechsler scale, have achieved general recognition. Tests of this kind take cognizance of arithmetical, verbal, and logical ability, and also other capacities such as the recognition of form. They roughly correspond, on the mental side of development, to the radiological atlases on the physical side; that is, certain test items represent the average attainment at the age of 9, others represent average performance at the age of 10, and so on. A child passing all the items in the group labelled 9 years, but failing all those in the next group, would be said to have a mental age of 9, irrespective of their chronological age. Special scoring methods allow intermediate estimates to be made in the case of children who may pass a proportion of items in the next higher group.

The mental age is thus an index of maturation of the mind, and, like the radiological age, increases at a rate which depends on many intrinsic and environmental factors. Thus, constant stimulation is required, the child being allowed the opportunity to develop problem-solving skills and to acquire other worldly experiences so as to prevent the risk of mental age becoming delayed in development. It is educationally sound to provide good teaching and interesting experiences wherever possible to encourage this mental capacity to increase more rapidly. Thus the interaction of external factors with internal growth and development is important to allow every child to attain their maximum potential. However, there is also the need for early recognition of problems which may interfere with normal mental development, such as dyslexia and other developmental anomalies so that appropriate remedial steps can be taken.

So little is known about mental processes that it is very difficult to say when mental development reaches maturity. A distinction must be made between non-verbal intelligence, which is tested by problems which do not require vocabulary or a store of information, and verbal intelligence, which depends on educational and environmental factors. Non-verbal intelligence appears to reach a maximum somewhere between 15 and 25 years of age, in conformity with the general growth of the body. Adverse factors such as a poor diet are important to recognize as they can affect the process. On the other hand, verbal intelligence can continue to increase until much later in life, depending on the circumstances of the individual. Mental capacity, measured by the tests in current use, deteriorates considerably in old age, partly because of the time limits imposed; given extra time, old people perform better than might be supposed.

A convenient way of classifying intelligence test performance is by the use of the concept of the 'Intelligence Quotient' (IQ), which is the mental age expressed as a percentage of the chronological age. Thus, a child with a mental age of 12 years and a chronological age of 10 would have an IQ of 120. Here again, as in the consideration of body size, it is difficult to satisfy the natural desire of administrators to separate off 'normal' from 'abnormal'. A child with an IQ of exactly 100 falls exactly in the middle of the 'standard' group from which the test was constructed, but what is to be made of children with an IQ of 80? Are they to be described as simply of lower than average intelligence, or are they abnormal? Again, it is difficult always to be sure that like is being compared with like; IQ tests formulated in one country are not necessarily applicable to another, or even to a different set of children in the same country.

The IQ is only a relative measure, not an absolute one, and it merely relates the performance of the child to that of a designated group of other children.The implications of a low IQ are not always easy to elucidate. There may be defects in memory, in language ability, in perception, or in grasp of abstract concepts. In Britain most university students have intelligence quotients of 120 or over on the revised Stanford-Binet scale, while those with intelligence quotients of 60 or less are usually not capable of coping with ordinary education.

The ability to draw a human figure is often used to assess development, and the items the child includes can be scored and rated in terms of mental age. There is good correlation between these scores and other assessments made between 5 and 11 years of age.

Another method of estimating mental development is simply to use as the standard the capacity of the child to read. A British survey of all children born in a given week in 1958 showed that by the time they had reached the age of 7 years several factors affecting the acquisition of skill in reading could be identified. For example, a child from socio-economic class V (unskilled manual workers) is 15 times more likely to be a non-reader at this age than a child from socio-economic class I (professional occupations). Those whose families live under poor or overcrowded housing conditions are behind those with no such handicap, and a child from a family of five or more children is about a year behind a child from a family of one or two.

A recent British investigation found that the body mass index was inversely associated with educational achievement, the highest prevalence of obesity being found in the least qualified.

Physiological age

A series of physiological and biochemical changes occur during growth. Some of these are directly related to the alteration in the size of the child: for example, the resting heart rate slows progressively from about 100 beats/min at the age of 2 years to the adult value of about 65–70 beats/min. This falls in with the general biological rule that the heart rate is inversely related to body size.

Similarly, the respiratory rate in a new-born infant can be as high as 40–45/min, compared with the adult rate of 12–16. Some physiological functions 'mature' much earlier than others. In early infancy the bile is dilute and the blood protein values are low, but both reach adult status within a few years. The filtration rate of the glomeruli of the kidney reaches its adult value by the age of about 2 or 3 years, but the blood pressure continues to rise, not only throughout the growth period, but also during the whole of adult life (the systolic pressure is about 80–88 mmHg at the age of 5 years, rising to the adult value of about 120 mmHg by the age of 18). The basal metabolic rate is highest in the new-born, and falls rapidly from 6 years to 20 years, with a more gradual fall throughout the rest of life. There is some doubt as to whether there is, or is not, a transient rise in the rate (or at least a failure to fall as expected) at the time of the adolescent spurt.

Many physiological and biochemical changes during growth show a sex difference in timing, for they are more closely related to other indices of maturation than to chronological age. Thus, girls show a spurt in systolic blood pressure which occurs earlier than the corresponding spurt in the male, and the resting mouth temperature, which falls by 0.5–1°C from infancy to maturity, reaches its adult value earlier in girls. The erythrocyte count and the blood volume of boys diverge away from the figures for girls at the time of the adolescent spurt.

In the plasma, inorganic phosphate shows a steady fall from the high levels of childhood to reach adult figures by the ages of 15 in girls and 17 in boys; the calcium level does not change during this period. The alkaline phosphatase rises significantly, in parallel with the growth velocity, between the ages of 8–12 in girls and 10–14 in boys; thereafter it falls rapidly to adult levels.

It has been suggested that some biochemical measurements might serve as an indication of physiological maturity, but there are considerable practical difficulties. Not only are there complications in measurement (for example, how does one define the 'resting state' in an infant 1 year old?), but there is so far a lack of the longitudinal studies which alone could provide a firm basis for such an assessment. It is known, for instance, that the affinity of haemoglobin for oxygen is greater in the new-born than in the adult, and there is a fall in this affinity between the ages of 2 and 15 years to values less than those of the adult, but as yet there is no firm evidence as to when the adolescent shift from 'low' to 'normal' values takes place. Perhaps a more promising index of maturity is the ratio of creatine to creatinine in the urine; this ratio is thought to fall progressively with age after about the age of $14\frac{1}{2}$ years, probably under hormonal influences. Girls maturing early have a lower ratio than those of the same chronological age maturing late, and a measurement of this ratio might be made to afford information regarding maturity if considered along with skeletal and other data obtained at the same time.

Late and early development

Six types of skeletal development have been recognized. There are first the average children, about whom little need be said. In the second group are children who are tall in childhood only because they have matured faster than average: they will not be particularly tall adults. The third group comprises those children who are not only early maturers, but who are genetically tall also. These children are taller than average from early childhood, and will be tall adults. The fourth group is the opposite of the second, and contains children who are small because they mature late, but who will eventually be of average stature; the fifth group is the opposite of the third, and is made up of those who are both late in developing and genetically short in stature. Finally, there is an indefinite group who start puberty either much earlier or much later than usual. As the 'growth life' of children in this category is longer or shorter than average, they may well turn out to be much taller or much shorter than would have been predicted.

It is probable that terminal stature is related more to the mean growth rate during the whole growing period than to the time of onset of the adolescent spurt or to the time at which closure of the epiphyses takes place.

The evidence suggests that mental and psychological development are much more closely linked with radiological and dental age than with chronological age, and that an individual classified as 'advanced' or 'retarded' physically will also be so classified mentally. Those who are quick to mature physically score better in intelligence tests than those of the same age who have not yet reached the same stage of physical development. The difference ceases to be detectable after full maturation of both groups.

Both the late and the early developers have their problems. For example, a boy who develops late may lag not only in height and weight, but also in motor skills and in the development of intelligence. As a result he does less well in school and in athletics, and may be 'kept back' in a lower class than that appropriate to his chronological age. As a consequence of this he is likely to feel rejected, and to be rebellious and aggressive, although his lack of muscular development renders him vulnerable in a fight. At the same time he is anxious about his failure to develop, and has a need for psychological support. It often can also create problems in employment, such as when an immature adolescent tries to join the Armed Forces.

Early maturation can also create difficulties for the child. To be physically bigger than one's colleagues is not necessarily an advantage when it comes to fitting in with the educational apparatus provided, and the attainment of an adult body and sexual maturity before the attainment of economic independence produces a situation which is aggravated by the increasing amounts of secondary and tertiary education demanded by modern civilization. In this respect, as in so many other features of modern life, it is more comfortable to conform.

6 Changes in shape and posture

By reason of the frailty of our nature we cannot always stand upright
Book of Common Prayer

The allometry equation

Just as the whole body grows at a varying rate from birth to maturity, so its component parts have their own rates of growth, which also change with age, although not necessarily synchronously. This leads to changes in bodily proportions. Occasionally, the relationship between the size of one part and the size of another, or between the size of one part and the whole body, can be described by a straight regression line; this argues that the relative growth rates of the two parts remain constant, and also that the difference between the two rates is established early in development.

But relations of this type may not always fit a simple linear regression, and differential growth is sometimes described by the so-called allometry equation.

$$y = bx^k$$

where y is the size of one part and x that of another, and b and k are constants. The form of the allometry equation implies that the part of the body studied grows at a rate which increases or decreases proportionately with time (unless k is unity). There is no good evidence for this, and if the equation is used to study such matters as the relation between sitting and standing heights, arm length and trunk length, and so on, it is found that after a certain age new values for b and k become necessary for most paired comparisons. In other words, the relationship between one part and another of the growing body is not a steady or consistent one, but changes with age. As an example, sitting height increases at adolescence much more rapidly than stature as a whole, whereas previous to adolescence it more or less keeps pace with stature.

D'Arcy Thompson developed the theory of transformations to deal with the changing shape of the body produced by differential growth of its components. The outline of the animal or part being studied is projected on to a system of Cartesian co-ordinates, which can then be deformed mathematically, perhaps by tilting the axes, or by locally altering the scale in some parts of the figure but not in others.

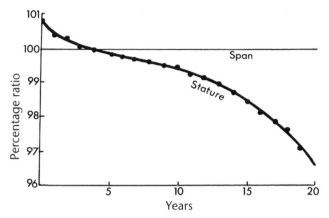

Fig. 6.1 Variations with age in the ratio of stature to the span of the out-stretched arms. Note that the ratio is still decreasing at the age of 20. (From Thompson, D'Arcy W. (1942). *Growth and form* (2nd edn). Cambridge University Press, London, by kind permission of the publishers.)

Shape of the infant

Because the head of the new-born baby is relatively very large the ratio of vertical head height to total height is $1:4$, whereas in the adult it is $1:7\frac{1}{2}$. This difference was not appreciated by many well-known early European painters, and it is common to find representations of the Virgin and Child in which the baby has the chubby outline typical of his age but the proportions typical of an adult. Again, because the lower limbs are poorly developed at birth they account for only about 15% of the total body weight, as compared with 30% in the adult, and the ratio of lower limb length to total height is $1:3$ in the new-born, but $1:2$ in the adult. This means that as growth proceeds there is a shift in the centre of gravity downwards, from about the level of the 12th thoracic vertebra in the infant to about the level of the fifth lumbar vertebra in the adult. As the child begins to walk before this shift has progressed very far, he is handicapped by being relatively top-heavy. At birth, the length of the foot is virtually the same as the length of the tibia, but in the adult it is only two-thirds as long. The span of the outstretched arms is less than the total height at birth, but rapidly overtakes it (Fig. 6.1). In a group of American white women at the stage of maximum height in their third decade, the span exceeded height by a mean of 1.8 cm. There are racial variations in these bodily proportions. For example, black Africans have relatively longer limbs, and their forearms and legs are longer relative to their arms and thighs than they are in the white races. Thus, the span of a group of black American women exceeded their maximum height by a mean of as much as 8.3 cm.

Because of the differential growth of the lower part of the body, the umbilicus, which at birth is 1–2 cm below the mid-point of the body, has reached the mid-point by the age of 1 year; in the adult it lies higher still, about 60% of the way up a line joining the heels to the top of the head.

The circumference of the skull at birth averages 33–36 cm, and this is about the same as the circumference of the chest: the circumference of the abdomen is greater than either until about the age of 2 years, because of the presence of the large liver and because the relatively small pelvis cannot contain several organs which are to be found in the adult pelvis, such as the urinary bladder (Fig. 4.10). The rapid development of the pelvis in early childhood allows the bladder and intestines to sink down into it, and this results in a flattening of the abdominal wall. The thorax, which, with the shoulder girdle, has been 'pushed up' towards the neck by the over-crowding in the abdomen, is allowed to descend, and there is thus an apparent lengthening of the neck, which is usually not visible in a well nourished baby, the chin and lower jaw being in contact with the chest and shoulders.

The shape of the infant determines some of the hazards of infancy. For example, the shortness of the neck makes it difficult and dangerous to perform a tracheostomy, for the left brachiocephalic vein may be pushed up above the suprasternal notch. The cross-section of the barrel-shaped infant chest is virtually circular, and remains so for the first 2 years; the ribs lie more or less horizontally. Thoracic respiration depends on being able to raise the ribs to a more horizontal position from a more vertical one, for their anatomy ensures that this manoeuvre will increase both the anteroposterior and the lateral diameters of the chest (Fig. 6.2). But if the ribs are already horizontal, it becomes impossible to increase the diameter of the chest by moving the ribs. It follows that the new-born baby has to depend almost completely on diaphragmatic breathing, and if an abdominal wound, such as a surgical operation, causes pain on movement of the abdominal wall, inadequate ventilation of the lungs may follow and pneumonia is a risk. Because the rib cage and sternum are higher than in the adult, the abdominal cavity of the infant is less well protected by bone.

Another anatomical danger lies in the fact that the external auditory meatus is poorly developed at birth. The ear drum is very close to the surface, and so is the facial nerve. Injury to the nerve may therefore be caused by obstetric forceps, and damage to the drum by unwary clinical examination.

The size of the infant in itself constitutes a danger. Like all small animals, a baby has a relatively large surface area, and the risk of losing or gaining heat is considerable. This is probably the reason for the plentiful supply of fat, which acts as an insulating agent between the internal organs and the outside world. At birth, the surface area of the head accounts for nearly 20% of that of the whole body (as opposed to about 7% in the adult), and is therefore a major portal of heat gain or loss. Because of the immaturity and inadequacy of the

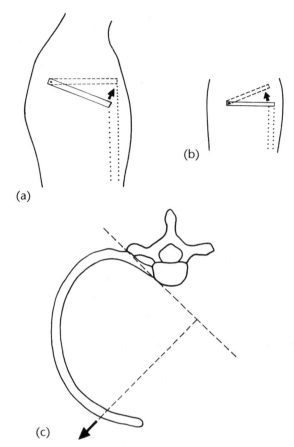

Fig. 6.2 Mechanics of respiration. (a) Diagram showing movement of adult rib. As the rib is raised, so the horizontal distance between its ends is increased, and thus the cavity of the chest enlarges until its size becomes maximal when the rib is horizontal. (b) In a baby's chest the rib is already horizontal. Further elevation of its anterior end decreases rather than increases the anteroposterior diameter of the chest. (c) Diagram to show that the motion of the anterior end of the rib is outwards as well as forwards. The rib articulates with the vertebra by two joints, one on the transverse process of the vertebra and one on the body, and rotates around a line drawn through these two joints. Its anterior end moves outwards and forwards in a direction at right angles to this line as the rib is raised to the horizontal, so enlarging the transverse as well as the anteroposterior diameter of the chest. Again, elevation of the horizontal rib in the baby cannot be effective in this way.

sweat glands the infant cannot adjust its temperature efficiently by sweating if it becomes overheated.

Changes in shape with growth

Figure 6.3 and Table 6.1 show the alterations which occur during growth in the

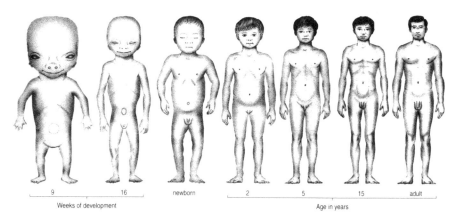

Fig. 6.3 Changes in body shape with age. Different parts of the human body grow at different rates. Note the relatively large head of the fetus at 9 weeks and, as the individual grows, how the other parts of the body grow much more than the head. (From Wolpert (1997), *Principles of Development*, OUP.)

proportions of the various parts of the body. At all ages the dimensions of the head are in advance of (i.e. nearer maturity than) those of the trunk, the trunk is in advance of the limbs, and the more peripheral parts of the limbs are in advance of the more central parts. Thus, the foot is nearer adult status than the calf, and the calf is more advanced than the thigh.

In the adolescent growth spurt, the feet and hands speed up first, then the calf and forearm, followed by the hips and chest, and then the shoulders. Last of all to accelerate are the length of the trunk and the depth of the chest; there is about a year between the peaks for lower limb length and trunk length. There is thus a transient stage during which the hands and feet are large and ungainly relative to the rest of the body, and this is sometimes a source of anatomical embarrassment to the adolescent. The spurt in trunk length is relatively greater than the spurt in the lower limbs, so that more of the increase in height at adolescence derives from the trunk than from the lower limbs. The foot stops growing early, before almost all other parts of the skeleton.

Table 6.1 Relative sizes of parts of the body

Age	Head and neck	Trunk	Upper limbs	Lower limbs
Birth	30	45	10	15
2 years	20	50	10	20
6 years	15	50	10	25
Adult	10	50	10	30

The figures are approximate percentages of total body volume.

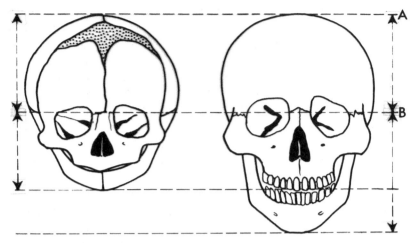

Fig. 6.4 Growth of the face. The newborn skull and the adult skull have been drawn so that the height of the cranial vault (the distance between the planes A and B) is the same. Notice the great relative increase in the facial skeleton in the adult. (See also Fig. 4.3.)

The bones of the face grow faster than those of the cranial vault, and it has been said that at adolescence the face 'emerges from under the skull' (Fig. 6.4). In infancy the main growth is in the jaws, which have to accommodate the teeth, but in adolescence the profile becomes straighter and the nose more projecting. All these changes are more noticeable in boys.

In adolescence, the shape of the face is also altered by changes in the hair. In the region of the frontal hairline, the terminal hairs are replaced by vellus in about 80% of females and in virtually every male, so causing a frontal recession of hair which may be progressive for several years. In the later stages of the adolescent spurt there is laterality of growth rather than a linearity, because the limb growth, which started first, exhausts itself first. The child who 'shoots up like a beanpole' proceeds to broaden in the later stages of adolescent spurt, and the clavicle, which thrusts the shoulder out from the trunk, is one of the last bones in the body to stop growing. Slow-maturing children tend to be long-legged and narrow hipped at maturity: fast maturing children become broader and more stocky.

During the adolescent spurt the sex differences in the skeleton become apparent; in the male the shoulders grow more than the pelvis, and in the female the reverse is true. The differential growth of the female pelvis, which causes it to become wider, shallower, and roomier than the male pelvis, is obviously related to the needs of childbearing, and the greater growth of the male shoulders is presumably related to the greater use of his more powerful muscles. But it is quite unknown how these changes are produced, although genetic and sex-hormone factors must be important.

Other differences between the male and female skeleton are present at birth, and are merely exaggerated at adolescence. For example, throughout the whole period of growth the male forearm is longer, relative to height, than the female forearm. Again, the female index finger is often as long as or longer than the ring finger, but this relationship is not so common in the male.

The deposition of fat in the female body at adolescence effects very considerable alterations in body shape (Fig. 3.1). There seems to be no good reason why the fat should be laid down at one place rather than at another, although the fat in the region of the breast clearly serves to protect the developing mammary gland. The process is under the control of the ovarian hormones, and administration of these hormones to a male will cause deposition of fat in the breast as well as development of mammary tissue. In the Bushmen and Hottentots of Africa there is a very marked accumulation of fat in the buttocks at the time of puberty; this is much more evident in the women than in the men, and is known as steatopygia. Nothing is known about its significance.

The accumulation of excess fat may produce alterations in the shape of other parts of the body. The increased weight may lead to flat feet or knock knees, or to an increase in the lumbar curvature of the vertebral column, a condition known as lordosis.

Classification of physique

People have different shapes as well as different sizes. It is possible to give mathematical expression to this fact by using the statistical technique of factor analysis, based on measurements made of various parts of the body. Such measurements may include total height, limb length, arm circumference, etc., and correlation coefficients can be derived from them. By factor analysis it is possible to account for much of the variability of the original measurements in terms of a smaller number of independent and more generalized factors. Such methods are as yet in their infancy, and, although they have a considerable potential value in research, they are not adequately descriptive of physique for the non-specialist.

Many attempts have been made to derive a meaningful classification of the variety of shapes presented by the human physique dating back to the time of Hippocrates in ancient Greece. The reason for this is that different physiques have been associated with different diseases and temperaments. The matter is therefore far from being a purely academic problem.

An early effort to describe physique mathematically was the Rohrer Index, an ancestor of the body mass index. This was 100 times the weight in grams divided by the cube of the height in centimetres. A figure of 1.0–1.15 indicated a slender build, one of 1.15—1.40 a medium build, and one of over 1.40 a heavy build. Another system depends on an 'androgyny rating'. This is a general assessment of the shape of the adult body in terms of sexual differences. For example, the male has a low and indefinite waist, whereas the female has a well marked one. The space between the legs in the male is relatively wide, and in the female is smaller. The distribution of body hair differs in the two sexes, and so does the amount of fat. These and other observations can be used to form a general rating system which gives some information regarding the shape of a given individual.

Even though these ratings are useful in a general way, they are not detailed enough to provide sufficient information for clinical and physiological conclusions to be reached. This difficulty was overcome in the 1920's and 1930's by the development of early systems to classify the body build visually and anthropometrically; these were later developed into the classical system known as 'somatotyping' by Sheldon and his collaborators in 1940.

Sheldon recognized three different components of physique. The first is 'endomorphy'. This describes the relative degree of fatness of the body, regardless of where or how it is distributed. An individual high in this component (an 'endomorph') is characteristically round. He has a round head, his abdomen is larger than his thorax, and his arms and thighs contain much fat, although his wrists and ankles are relatively thin. He has large viscera, and a good deal of subcutaneous fat. His body measures more from front to back than from side to side.

The second component is 'mesomorphy' which describes the relative musculoskeletal development of the body. A 'mesomorph' has strong and robust shoulders and chest, a transversely lying heart, and heavily muscled limbs: the forearms and calves are relatively stronger than the arms and thighs. He has little subcutaneous fat and is thicker from side to side than from front to back.

The third component of the somatotype is called ectomorphy and describes the relative slenderness of the body. An 'ectomorph' is thin, stretched-out and narrow, with little muscle, little subcutaneous fat, and thin limbs. The heart lies vertically, and both the skin surface and the nervous system are relatively large. The adolescent spurt takes place about a year later than that of a typical mesomorph.

Sheldon found it possible to recognize the relative contributions to each of these three components of physique in any given individual, and so to record his 'somatotype'. By using a special photographic technique, he developed a subjective scoring system in which each component was allotted a mark on a rigid scale of 1—7 arbitrary units.

However, the original method as devised by Sheldon has shortcomings, mainly as it relies on a use of a rigid closed seven-point scale combined with a lack of objectivity in the application of the ratings. In response to these

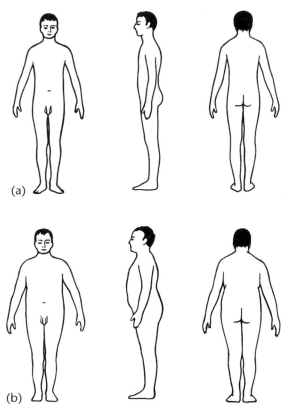

Fig. 6.5 Somatotypes. (a) An average individual, showing even balance between the three components. (Somatotype 4-3$\frac{1}{2}$-4.) (b) Predominant endomorphy, with minimal admixture of the other components. (Somatotype 7-1-1$\frac{1}{2}$.) (Based on photographs in Sheldon, W. H. and Stevens. S. S. (1942). *The varieties of temperament*. Harper and Row, New York, by kind permission of the authors.)

problems, a new method emerged with open rating scales, objective ratings and a phenotypic approach. This is called the Heath–Carter somatotype method and is now the most universally employed method in human biology.

Somatotyping gives an overall summary of the physique as a unified whole and tells you what sort of physique you have and how it looks. It has been found to be of great value in describing and comparing the physiques of athletes in a variety of sports and at all levels as well as the changes that occur during growth, ageing, training, and physical performance.

Applying somatotyping to a person in whom ectomorphy predominates to an extreme degree, a score would be recorded as 1 1 7, whereas an extreme endomorph would be written 7-1-1. These unusual somatotypes are extremes of the normal, as most people are usually classified at about 4-3-3 or 3-4-4 (Figs. 6.5 and 6.6). It is remarkable that with such apparently vague and subjective criteria, different observers, if properly experienced, vary by only

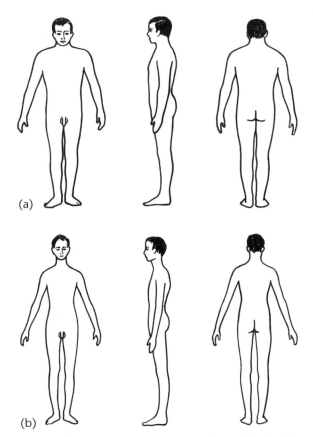

(a)

(b)

Fig. 6.6 Somatotypes. (a) Predominant mesomorphy, with minimal admixture of the other components (Somatotype 1-7-1$\frac{1}{2}$). (b) Predominant ectomorphy, with minimal admixture of the other components. (Somatotype 1$\frac{1}{2}$-1$\frac{1}{2}$-7.) (Based on photographs in Sheldon, W. H. and Stevens, S. S. (1942). *The varieties of temperament*. Harper and Row, New York, by kind permission of the authors.)

about half a mark in the analysis of each individual.

Difficulties are introduced into the statistical handling of somatotype data by the fact that the three components are not independent of each other, so that certain theoretically possible somatotypes are not found in practice. Thus there are no people who can be written 7-7-1 or 7-3-6, to take only two of many such examples.

The normal age for taking the somatotype is 20–25 years, and it is believed to remain constant throughout adult life. With the passage of years, an individual may put on or lose fat, increase the size of his muscles by training, or allow them to atrophy from disuse. Nevertheless, it is claimed that a trained somatotyper can penetrate the various changes a person might make in this way to their basic external form.

Most of the work on somatotyping has been done with males, but women also show a similar range of physique. The distribution of somatotypes is, however, somewhat different, for mesomorphic build is relatively much rarer in females than in males. The difference may be in part genetic, and in part because the muscular development dependent on testosterone does not usually take place.

Certain facts have accumulated regarding the relationship of body form measured in this way to physical, psychological, and physiological differences. For example, endomorphs more readily put on fat in middle age, and are more prone to develop a late-onset diabetes than an early-onset diabetes. Ectomorphs have short reaction times to external stimuli, and are liable to tuberculosis. Mesomorphs have a high blood volume, and commonly suffer from coronary disease.

The reasons behind such empirical observations indicate a fascinating line of research. Studies in Africa have shown that the warmer the environment the lower is the body weight relative to height and the longer are the limbs relative to the trunk. Under the warmest conditions, physique tends to become linear, as in the Dinkas who have limbs which are narrow and elongated (particularly the forearms and legs), a short trunk, and little subcutaneous fat. Whether this physique results from genetic, nutritional, or physiological influences is not yet established, but people with a linear build have a greater surface area than endomorphs or mesomorphs of similar body weight. It is therefore at least possible that the linearity of the Dinkas represents to some extent an evolutionary adaptation.

Sheldon and Stevens also analysed personality in exactly the same way as physique by describing three components of temperament; each of these was defined by 20 traits, which are shown in Table 6.2. Each trait was scored on a scale from 1 to 7, and the trait score was then averaged to get the rating for each component. When the personality ratings of a series of subjects were compared with their somatotypes, significant correlations (about 0.8) were obtained between 'viscerotonia' and endomorphy, 'somatotonia' and mesomorphy, and 'cerebrotonia' and ectomorphy.

Other studies have dealt with the effect of body type on choice of career. It is not unexpected to find that mesomorphs choose careers consistent with their athletic build such as physical training instructors, army officers, and so on. But it has also been found that workers on the research side of a factory at all levels were more ectomorphic than those who were concerned with production in the same factory. In another investigation, students of engineering, medicine, and dentistry were found to be more mesomorphic than students of physics and chemistry, who tended to be more ectomorphic. Yet again, it appears that juvenile delinquents tend to be mesomorphic. Others have related different kinds of psychiatric disturbance to body build. Anxiety states seem to be more

Table 6.2 Personality traits

Viscerotonia	Somatotonia	Cerebrotonia
*1. Relaxation in posture and movement	*1. Assertiveness of posture and movement	*1. Restraint in posture and movement; tightness
*2. Love of physical comfort	*2. Love of physical adventure	2. Physiological over-response
*3. Slow reaction	*3. The energetic characteristic	3. Overly fast reactions
*4. Love of eating	*4. Need and enjoyment of exercise	*4. Love of privacy
*5. Socialization of eating	5. Love of dominating, lust for power	*5. Mental overintensity, hyperattentionality. Apprehensiveness
6. Pleasure in digestion	6. Love of risk and chance	*6. Secretiveness of feeling, emotional restraint
*7. Love of polite ceremony	*7. Bold directness of manner	*7. Self-conscious motility of the eyes and face
*8. Sociophilia	*8. Physical courage for combat	*8. Sociophobia
*9. Indiscriminate amiability	*9. Competitive aggressiveness	*9. Inhibited social address
10. Greed for affection and approval	10. Psychological callousness	10. Resistance to habit and poor routinizing
11. Orientation to people	11. Claustrophobia	11. Agoraphobia
*12. Evenness of emotional flow	12. Ruthlessness, freedom from squeamishness	12. Unpredictability of attitude
*13. Tolerance	*13. The unrestrained voice	*13. Vocal restraint, and general restraint of noise
*14. Complacency	14. Spartan indifference to pain	14. Hypersensitivity to pain
15. Deep sleep	15. General noisiness	15. Poor sleep habits, chronic fatigue
*16. The untempered characteristic	*16. Overmaturity of appearance	*16. Youthful intentness of manner and appearance
*17. Smooth, easy communication of feeling, extraversion of viscerotonia	17. Horizontal mental cleavage, extraversion of somatotonia	17. Vertical mental cleavage, introversion
18. Relaxation and sociophilia under alcohol	18. Assertiveness and aggression under alcohol	18. Resistance to alcohol, and to other depressant drugs
19. Need of people when troubled	19. Need of action when troubled	19. Need of solitude when troubled
20. Orientation toward childhood and family relationships	20. Orientation toward goals and activities of youth	20. Orientation toward the later periods of life

Note. The 30 traits asterisked constitute collectively the short form of the scale. The table is reproduced from Sheldon, W. H. and Stevens, S. S. (1942). *The varieties of temperament.* Harper and Row, New York, by kind permission of the authors.

common in ectomorphs, although hysteria and depression are commoner in those with high scores in endomorphy and mesomorphy. Manic-depressive conditions tend to occur in people high in endomorphy and mesomorphy, but ectomorphs suffer from schizophrenia. There seems to be a pretty fair share-out of trouble all round!

It would clearly be important if we could predict the adult somatotype by means of information derived from measurements of the child.

There are difficulties with somatotype classification of children with accuracy, mainly as there are inadequate amounts of data which describe transformations in body shape with age during the period of growth.

Changes in posture with growth

The adult vertebral column has sagittal curvatures in the cervical, thoracic, lumbar, and pelvic regions. However, in contrast, the new-born infant has only two curvatures which are the consequence of the embryo developing in a position of flexion within the mother's uterus. These curves are both concave forwards, one being in the thoracic region, and the other being in the pelvis, formed by the curve of the sacrum which at this stage consists of separate sacral vertebrae. (Figs. 6.7 and 6.8). As growth of the infant occurs, the sacral curvature becomes permanently fixed by the fusing together of its vertebral components; the thoracic curve allows a certain limited amount of movement, but the intervertebral discs in this region are thin, and this restricts the scope of movement of one vertebra on another; movement is also limited by the oblique set of the spines of the vertebrae and the fact that their laminae overlap each other.

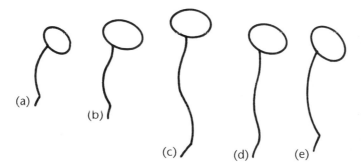

Fig. 6.7 Changes in the spinal curvatures with growth.
(a) Infant. Two primary curvatures.
(b) Six months, The secondary cervical curvature has appeared.
(c) Adult. Two primary and two secondary curvatures.
(d) Old age. The two secondary curvatures, dependent on the discs and the postural muscles, are becoming obliterated.
(e) Final stage, corresponding to condition in infant.

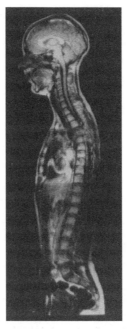

Fig. 6.8 MRI image taken through the midline of an adult. Note the presence of the spinal curvatures in the neck, thorax, abdomen and pelvic regions of the vertebral column. The image is a composite of three separate scans edited together using special computer software.

Prenatal functional muscle development leads to the appearance of a secondary curve in the cervical region of the column which becomes more pronounced at about 3 months of age when the baby begins to hold its head up (Fig. 6.9). This curvature, unlike the two primary ones, is convex forwards, and remains mobile, for its radius depends on the tension of the muscles which stretch across its concavity. The mobility of the cervical curvature is largely due to the thick intervertebral discs, which allow considerable 'play' between one vertebra and its neighbours.

On top of this secondary curvature, the skull has to be held balanced. At birth the position on the skull of the facets which articulate with the atlas vertebra is similar in all anthropoids. In apes the portion of the base of the skull in front of the joint grows more than the portion behind, so that the joint shifts backwards and the centre of gravity of the skull and brain is placed well forward. In humans there is much less discrepancy between the growth of the skull in front of the joint and behind it. The result is that the joint comes to lie relatively much further forwards than in the apes, although the centre of gravity of the head is still in front of it. The skull therefore balances reasonably well on top of the vertebral column, but it still requires some muscular effort to keep the gaze horizontal.

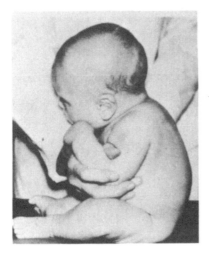

Age 8 weeks. Back rounded, raising head well.

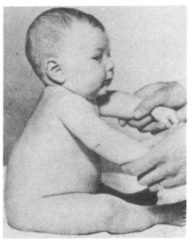

Age 16 weeks. Back straighter.

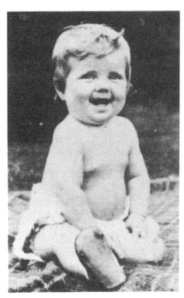

Age 26 weeks. Sitting, supported by hands.

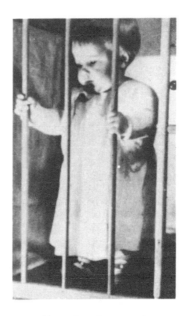

Age 52 weeks. Can stand, supported by furniture, and can walk, holding on to it ('cruises').

Fig. 6.9 Development of posture during first year of life. (From Illingworth, R. S. (1987). *The development of the infant and young child* (9th edn). Churchill Livingstone, London, by kind permission of the author and the publishers.)

When the baby begins to sit up at about 9 months (Fig. 6.9), the lumbar curvature appears, exaggerating a pre-existing lumbar flattening which was present during fetal development. This secondary curvature is also convex forwards like the cervical one. It is mobile, depending largely on the discs rather than on the shape of the bones for its evolution and is controlled by the great postural muscles of the vertebral column (Fig. 6.7).

Finally, the infant commences walking at about 12–15 months. All these functional changes of the first 18 months of life combine to exert a major influence on the development of the secondary curvatures in the vertebral column and also result in marked changes in the proportional size of the vertebra, especially in the lumbar region.

Both the secondary curvatures often fail to develop at the expected time if there is any delay in the development of the postures of sitting and holding the head up.

At the creeping stage, the baby is essentially a four-footed animal, albeit with exceptionally mobile forelimbs, and its centre of gravity is supported in a very stable manner by the quadrupedal posture. When this quadruped rears itself up on to its feet for its first efforts in walking (Fig. 6.9), it has an awkward and unstable stance. Because the centre of gravity is high, the infant must stand with legs held widely apart in order to maintain a secure balance. As the centre of gravity also lies well forward, partly because of the large liver, there is a compensatory exaggeration of the lumbar curvature in order to bring the upper part of the body into the vertical position; this usually ceases to be necessary about the age of 4 years. In the early stages of walking the baby is

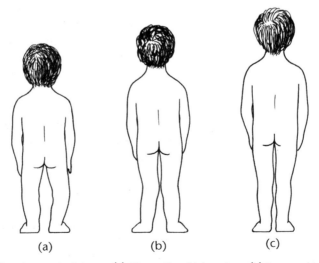

Fig. 6.10 Development of stance. (a) 18 months old: bow legs; (b) 3 years old: knock knees; (c) 6 years old: legs straight.

often bow-legged (Fig. 6.10); this corrects itself gradually, and may be followed by a knock-kneed period. About the age of $3-3\frac{1}{2}$ years, 75% of children have a distance of more than 2.5 cm between their medial malleoli, and in over 20% the distance is 5 cm or more. The condition usually rectifies itself by the age of 7 years. As the baby stands up, so the weight of the body pressing down on the lumbosacral joint forces the upper part of the sacrum forwards and downwards so that its lower portion and the coccyx are restrained by the sacrotuberous and sacrospinous ligaments from rotating upwards in consequence of this, with the result that the sacrum sinks more deeply in between the two hip bones. As the legs straighten and the weight is transmitted to the heads of the femora, the pelvis becomes steadily remodelled and the force which is applied to the sacrum tends to lever outwards the walls of the pelvic cavity, broadening the region of the symphysis and increasing the subpubic angle. The acetabula become deeper and the hip joints more stable as the child becomes more active in his newly acquired two-legged freedom.

In the new-born baby, the hips and knees are flexed and the feet are inverted; as walking begins, the lower limbs straighten out and the feet evert, and at the same time the angle made by the neck of the femur with the shaft decreases gradually from about 160° to the adult value of approximately 125°. The shaft of the infant femur is straight, and the forward curve characteristic of the adult bone begins to appear as the child stands up.

In the adult the centre of gravity is at about 55% of the total height from the floor, being higher in men than in women. The line of gravity drawn through it naturally alters constantly according to posture. When the subject is standing at rest the line normally falls behind the hip, in front of the ankle, and half-way between the heel and the balls of the toes (Fig. 6.11). It passes in front of the dens of the axis vertebra, the front of the body of the second thoracic vertebra, the middle of the body of the twelfth thoracic vertebra, and the back of the body of the fifth lumbar vertebra (Fig. 6.12). If the centre of gravity is allowed to fall too far backwards or forwards, muscular effort is needed to prevent falling.

A most important factor in posture is the tilt of the pelvis in relation to the horizontal. This is measured by the angle with the horizontal made by a line through the sacral promontory and the upper border of the symphysis pubis (Fig. 6.12), which is normally about 60°. The pelvic tilt is determined by the postural pull of the muscles of the back, abdomen, and thighs, and these pulls are in turn influenced by the way the individual habitually stands. A 'tense' habit of standing increases the tilt, so that the pelvis rotates forwards on the thighs, carrying the lumbar spine forwards, and with it the centre of gravity. In compensation, the upper part of the body is thrust backwards, so increasing the lumbar curvature. The neck is held stiffly, with the chin tucked in, in order to maintain the horizontal gaze of the eyes. If this posture is held as a routine,

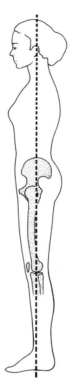

Fig. 6.11 Position of line of gravity in erect posture. The line passes through the external auditory meatus, the tip of the acromion process of the scapula, and the mid-point between the heel and the balls of the toes. It falls behind the hip joint, through the middle of the knee joint, and in front of the ankle joint.

the muscles which have pulled the pelvis out of position may shorten and their opponents lengthen, so that after a time the individual is unable to stand in any other way.

The converse of the 'tense' posture is the 'slack' posture. The pelvic tilt decreases, the centre of gravity passes backwards, and the head and thorax are thrust forwards to compensate. There is thus a mild increase in the thoracic curvature, and the neck is extended, the chin being poked forwards. The joints of the lower limb tend to flex, and become mechanically unstable.

Poor posture results from many causes, which are not always as easy to determine as might be thought. The damage may originate in any part of the body, for posture is an integral whole, and anything that tends to upset one part of the mechanism will throw the rest out of gear. A good example is the very common defect known as 'round shoulders', in which the muscles fail to hold the scapulae back towards the spine, so that the whole shoulder girdle drifts round the side of the chest towards the front of the body. Arm weight in

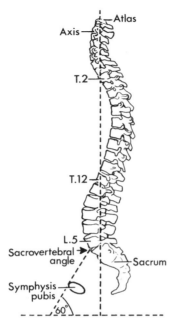

Atlas

Axis

T.2

T.12

L.5

Sacrovertebral angle

Symphysis pubis

Sacrum

60°

Fig. 6.12 The line of gravity in relation to the vertebral column. The pelvic tilt is usually about 60° (see text).

front of the gravity line has to be compensated for by alterations in the curvatures of the spine, and this in turn causes a movement of the pelvis which has repercussions on the posture of the joints of the lower limb and on the distribution of weight in the foot.

The wearing of high-heeled shoes, which tip the body weight forwards, can lead to disturbances of the posture of the whole body, working upwards through the pelvis to the spine; a complaint of aching pain in the neck can sometimes be cured by wearing a lower heel.

Postural deformities can be caused by injury or disease, but there is also a hereditary factor, and mental attitudes are also of importance in determining how the child 'holds himself'. Deformities commonly develop in adolescence, when the rapid increase in weight of the skeleton and body structures may not be accompanied for some time by a corresponding increase in the strength of the postural muscles, especially in girls. Those people who have six lumbar vertebrae instead of five have a greater part of their spinal column unprotected by the leverage of the rib cage, and tend to have trouble in this region.

Abnormal curvature of the vertebral column, called scoliosis, can seriously affect posture and body shape. This is a curvature of the bones of the vertebral column in which a twisting deformity bends the bones to one side, especially in the thoracic region, producing a marked hump prominence in the back in more severe cases. Some of these curvature deformities can result from sporting activities such as the minor curvatures of the vertebral column often encountered in tennis players and discus throwers. Others occur as a result of leg length inequality or developmental abnormalities in the bones of the vertebral column. Perhaps the most distressing cases are the severe scolioses which occur in adolescent girls at about puberty where the cause is probably due to a combination of growth factors and an as yet unknown developmental abnormality which affects the nervous system.

Drawbacks of the erect posture

Standing in the erect position has brought certain advantages with it to humans. The hands are freed, allowing manipulation of objects and coordination between the hands and the brain. This in turn is responsible for an increase in the size of the brain, and for our capacity to make and use tools. A second advantage is that the eyes are brought further from the ground and made more mobile, as the skull can now be poised more freely on the top of the vertebral column.

But the erect posture also brings with it many disabilities, some of which are apparent quite early in life, while others arise later, when the pull of gravity and the effects of tissue degeneration have been operating for a long time.

In the first place, a great part of the large central nervous system has to be devoted to maintaining the precarious equilibrium by a complex system of reflexes and controls. Proprioception or position sense is a vital component of this mechanism. The loss of these control mechanisms following viral illness, which can attack particular nerve tracts or nerve fibres, or in old age, is severely debilitating and can leave a sufferer bed-bound and entirely reliant on medical support. Secondly, there is an increased burden on the bones and joints of the lower limb, particularly on the foot, which leads to flat feet, sprained ankles, etc. These are much in evidence following the adolescent growth spurt, when violent exercise may throw an intolerable strain on the ankle region, and when periods of prolonged standing at work may place too much gravitational load on the arches of the feet.

There is also a considerable strain on the cantilever structure of the vertebral column, which is not yet fully adapted by evolution to being tipped up on end (Fig. 6.13). Aches and pains, degenerating joints, and damage to intervertebral discs are all common in the lower part of the column.

The pelvis remains essentially the pelvis of a four-footed animal, but it has to continue to allow the passage of the fetal skull, which in the course of evolution has grown bigger, while at the same time coping with a very large gravitational strain. This mechanical problem is aggravated by the postural

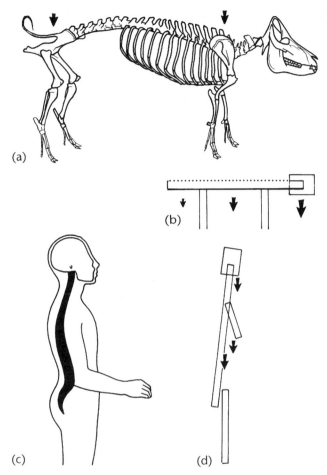

Fig. 6.13 Stresses in the vertebral column (a) Skeleton of a pig: the arrows indicate the points at which weight is transferred to the limbs. (b) Compare with the plan of a two-armed centilever. The solid line indicates compression forces taken by the bones, the dotted line indicates tension forces. The spines of the vertebrae in (a) are long and powerful in order to afford attachment to muscles and ligaments resisting tension forces. (c) and (d) When this structure is stood on end, the stresses which it has to withstand are quite different.

burden which a heavy pregnant uterus lying in front of the line of gravity imposes on the vertebral column, and women who have borne several children may have troublesome pain in the lower part of the back resulting from the stress laid upon their lumbosacral and sacroiliac joints.

In the upright position, the forelimbs hang down at the side of the trunk at right angles to their former 'neutral' position. The resulting extensive anatomical alterations in the shoulder region have made some of the nerves and vessels entering the limb liable to compression and injury.

Breathing is hampered, as the weight of the chest wall must be raised against the pull of gravity instead of swinging at right angles to it, as in the four-footed animal. The rib cage therefore falls in old age, when the muscles are no longer equal to the heavy task of raising it in inspiration; the result is deficient ventilation. The thoracic and abdominal viscera descend, and the anterior abdominal wall becomes weakened because of increased pressure on the lower portion of it; this is a factor in the frequency of hernia. Similarly, there is an increased gravitational load on the pelvic floor, which shows itself in the frequency of the condition of prolapse, in which the uterus and bladder descend through a pelvic diaphragm weakened or damaged by childbirth.

Finally, the elevation of the brain above the heart means that gravity interferes with its blood supply. The return of blood to the heart from the lower limbs is also impeded by the long vertical haul against gravity. For this reason, the autonomic nervous system has had to develop a complicated system of vasomotor controls, and these are not always adequate to the occasion, as is seen in the condition of postural fainting, in which the blood supply to the brain is interrupted when the patient suddenly stands up. The common condition of varicose veins also testifies to the incomplete adaptation of the vascular system.

The erect posture is therefore not an unmixed blessing, and the gradual achievement of it during the first part of childhood carries with it liabilities as well as advantages. In old age, many of these liabilities come home to roost, and posture undergoes regressive changes which will be dealt with in Chapter 11.

7 Genetic and hormonal factors influencing growth and maturation

Boy (20), 5 ft. 7 ins., wishes to increase height to 5 ft. 10 ins.
The Times, 6 November 1968

Genetic control

Although the growth of the individual is the result of a complex interaction of many different factors, which include genetic and environmental influences, it is clear that the genetic component of the individual and what they inherit from their parents is a powerful factor in how they progress through life (Fig. 7.1). For example, the best way of growing tall and heavy is to have tall and heavy parents, while studies of twins have shown that body shape and size, deposition of fat, and patterns of growth, are all more nearly related to a genetic influence rather than to external factors.

Your genes not only influence your own individual size. Genes also govern the anatomical differences between all humans and our near relatives the chimpanzee and other primates. Evolution over time has allowed small mutations and selective forces to work on our species, determining our present anatomical form and body shape, which as a consequence is very different from that of our common ancestor (Chapter 6). Furthermore, this genetic process also influences and determines why we take a relatively long time to reach adulthood compared with other animals by controlling the rate at which we grow and mature. Thus the radiological, dental, sexual, and neurological ages (Chapter 5) of identical twins tend also to be identical, whereas those of non-identical twins may differ considerably.

Although the overall control of body size is complex and involves many genes, a disturbance in a single gene or group of genes can produce widespread and drastic effects, such as in the condition of achondroplasia, which is inherited as a simple dominant.

However, the effects of genetic control are often quite restricted and specific. For example, the genetic control of dental maturation and eruption appears to be separate from that of skeletal maturation, and there is evidence that the genes controlling the growth of different segments of the limbs are

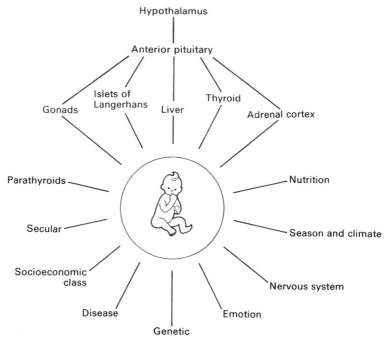

Fig. 7.1 Factors affecting growth.

independent of each other. It is now believed that dental development and the sequence of ossification are primarily genetically controlled; the timing of ossification is partly influenced by genetic factors and partly by environmental ones. Maturation as a whole is even more affected by environment, but genetic influences are still detectable.

Certain groups of people are taller than others. In Africa, the Dinkas and Watsui are one of the tallest races, and the Mubuti and other pygmies of Central Africa among the smallest. It is probable that evolution and genetic factors are largely responsible for such racial differences, although nutrition must also play an important part. It is now established that, at least in Central African pygmies, while the secretion of growth hormone (hGH) by the pituitary is normal in quantity, and the same in chemical composition, insulin-like growth factor 1 (IGF-1) levels are in fact lower. This suggests that there may be a genetic defect which affects the production of the IGF-1. Similar findings have been reported in miniature breeds of dog such as the poodle. The presumed genetic effect which keeps them small must therefore influence the tissues upon which the hormonal control acts, rendering them in some way unresponsive and failing to produce the IGF-1 at normal amounts. Certainly, experimental injection of hGH into pygmies produces none of the usual biochemical changes associated with such injections in other races. Interestingly, in a study of height in the Twa (Pygmies), the tallest Twa was found to have a height greater than the smallest Tutsi who live in nearby Central Africa.

There are racial differences in skeletal maturation. African children in West Africa and East Africa and Afro-Caribbeans in the United States are ahead of white children living in these areas at birth, and for the first year or two they grow faster. They are also ahead in functional stages of development such as sitting up and crawling (Table 5.2).

However, the growth curves are different in the two races, so that by about the fourth year the initial difference in growth has been abolished and the skeletal advancement, together with the advancement in performance tests, has disappeared. This might possibly be because by the third year the effects of inadequate nutrition have neutralized the racial or genetic advantage of the black children. But the permanent teeth also erupt about a year earlier in black people than in white, although by this time the effects of nutrition would certainly be operative.

A racial factor is involved in the mineral content of bone. A high bone density is common among African races, and the bones of Polynesian women are denser than those of European women living alongside them in New Zealand. These racial differences may be of importance in relation to osteoporosis. It is often supposed that the differences in average height between Eastern and European races are due to earlier closure of the epiphyses of the long bones in the former, but work in India and elsewhere has shown that there is insufficient evidence for this conclusion, and that these differences are probably due to differences in average growth per annum during the whole growing period, genetically determined, and modified by nutritional factors.

It would be interesting to have observations on the skeletal maturation and epiphyseal closure of groups of people who are naturally small, such as the pygmies in Central Africa, but the major difficulty in such an investigation still remains of establishing accurate chronological ages of the subjects. Study of tribes of small size in New Guinea may possibly supply such information.

Genetic factors are clearly important in determining the difference between male and female patterns of growth. As regards size, there is little to choose between boys and girls up to the age of 10 years, although boys are on the average slightly heavier at birth. Although recent allometry and growth studies underline the fact that subtle changes are present between the sexes, even at birth, it is the timing and intensity of the adolescent growth spurt which is responsible for the size difference between adult men and women. The onset of this spurt is mainly genetically controlled, although its intensity and duration probably depend on hormonal factors and can also be affected by environmental factors.

The advancement of girls over boys in respect of skeletal maturation has been attributed to a retarding action of the genes on the Y chromosome of the male. Individuals with the sex chromosome complement XXY (approximately

2 in 1000 new-born males) suffer from Klinefelter's syndrome; they are long-legged, show some enlargement of the breasts, and have grossly deficient spermatogenesis. Yet their skeletal retardation approximates that of normal males, despite their possession of two X chromosomes, which, it might be imagined, would tend to produce a female pattern of maturation. The onset of puberty is not delayed, but its progress is slow. There are usually some difficulties with education, as verbal intelligence is mildly affected.

Females with one instead of two X chromosomes (Turner's syndrome) have rudimentary or absent ovaries and lack secondary sexual characteristics. Such individuals suffer from short stature. They are plotted below the third centile of height, both as children and as adults, and do not grow to more than about 152 cm tall. The adolescent spurt does not occur, and the growth rate may actually decrease instead. Congenital deformities are common, but there is no mental handicap. Turner's syndrome is found in about 1 in 2000 live births, although it is much more common in the fetus; the disparity is accounted for by a high rate of fetal death. Treatment of Turner's syndrome with oestrogens ensures the development of female adult characteristics such as the breasts and hGH replacement therapy can add between 5 and 10 cm to the final height, correcting some of the effects of short stature.

Individuals with the pattern XYY (about 1.5 in 1000 new-born males) tend to be tall, but it is often difficult to track their skeletal maturation due to ethical problems associated with repeated radiographs of such individuals. This appears to be the only sex chromosomal abnormality in which there is no interference with growth. An investigation of over 4000 men more than 184 cm tall in Copenhagen found that 12 had the pattern XYY and 16 the pattern XXY.

Finally, about 1 in 25 000 males possesses the female pattern of two X chromosomes. Such XX men have normal male genitalia, but small testes: there is no production of spermatozoa.

The abnormal complement of sex chromosomes encountered in these different syndromes can often be very complex due to the existence of mosaicism where some cells in the body display one abnormal number of sex chromosomes while other cells possess a different complement. The overall effect of this problem is difficult to elicit and is still being actively researched.

Neural control

It has been suggested that there may be a 'growth centre' in the brain, possibly in the hypothalamus, and that this is responsible for keeping the child on his genetically determined growth curve wherever possible. If he deviates from this curve for any reason, such as malnutrition or illness, a period of accelerated 'catch-up' growth ensues. This phenomenon implies some sort of central control mechanism, and the reason for locating the hypothetical 'growth centre' in the hypothalamus is that the hypothalamus interacts with the anterior lobe of the pituitary gland in one of the basic hormonal controls of growth. There is also evidence that the peripheral nervous system plays some part in the control of growth. If somatic muscle is denervated, it atrophies, and, similarly, taste buds deprived of their innervation will degenerate. When a nerve supplying the hand or foot is cut, the growth of the nails within its territory is retarded in comparison with that of the nails supplied by other nerves, and returns to normal with the regeneration of the nerve. These effects and others like them are not sufficiently explained by the disuse following the injury or by a diminution in blood flow consequent on this disuse. It is therefore believed that the peripheral nerve fibres exert a nutritive or 'trophic' effect on the structures they supply, by means of a chemical secreted by the nerve cells and liberated at the nerve terminals; this substance modifies the growth and repair pattern of the structures innervated. Sensory nerve fibres exert a rather greater stimulating effect than motor fibres. The substance involved is probably not a normal neural transmitter but one of the many different local cytokine or other growth promoting agents which have been discovered. It is relevant to note that regeneration of a limb in animals which are capable of this feat depends, in its early stages at any rate, on the presence of an intact and sufficiently dense sensory nerve supply to the stump.

Finally, there is the question of central pattern generators. These are said to be pre-existing in-built patterns held within the nervous system which determine the growth and development of the limbs and peripheral parts of the body. Such a mechanism implies that in-built neural shape maps are mediated and put in place by local growth factors to ensure normal growth of the tissues concerned.

Local control

The growth of cells, and thus of tissues, depends on a complex interaction of local or regional influences. These paracrine factors include proteins which act as signalling factors, local growth factors, and the inhibitory control mechanisms of chalones and other substances. Adjacent cells may affect growth, either by contact or by a chemical stimulus, and cells of adjacent tissues may also control growth by chemical products. The autocrine chain of mechanisms allowing growth factors and hormones to enter the cell and affect the nucleus can go wrong with disastrous results. Finally, the age of a tissue has an important bearing on the amount of mitosis it can undertake.

Hormonal control

It is almost certain that all the endocrine glands influence growth. However, in the fetus, hormones can play no part in growth control before the end of the second month of fetal life, for until about this time the glands to elaborate them have not been formed. In this instance local acting growth promoters play a major part in regulating the growth of individual cells, aided by the genetic factors within the cell, which govern its responses to these agents. Furthermore, these agents almost certainly continue to play a part in growth after the development and commencement of function by the endocrine glands. As described earlier, the maximum rate of growth in height occurs about the fourth month of fetal life, and by this time the pituitary and thyroid glands are certainly functional.

The gonads apparently play no part in fetal growth, and the activity of the parathyroids is uncertain. The role of the fetal suprarenal cortex is not yet fully established. However, it appears that the pars intermedia of the pituitary gland is responsible for breaking down adrenocorticotrophic hormone (ACTH) produced by the anterior lobe into a fraction which stimulates the fetal cortex to produce growth-stimulating androgens rather than corticosteroids. Towards birth, the pars intermedia becomes less active, the fetal cortex decreases in size, and the production of androgens falls while that of corticosteroids rises. It is therefore possible that this mechanism plays an important part in growth before birth.

Growth hormone

The anterior lobe of the pituitary gland produces the polypeptide growth hormone (referred to as human growth hormone or hGH), which exists in two principal forms and several other forms in small amounts in the circulation. The difference between the two principal forms relates to their size, one with a molecular weight of 22 000 and the other of 20 000, and activity, with the smaller form appearing to have less action on carbohydrate metabolism. Human chromosome 17 has been found to contain five genes, one of which, hGN-N, codes for the most abundant form of hGH. The smaller form of hGH appears in appreciable amounts during pregnancy, although the reason for this is unclear. Its controlling gene is hGH-V which is expressed by the placenta. hGH can be detected in the body of the fetus as early as the end of the second month, very soon after the pituitary has been formed.

hGH is not essential for the growth of the fetus, for the bodies of anencephalic children, in whom the pituitary fails to develop, are of normal size. It was formerly thought that children deficient in hGH could not be identified for several years after birth, as their growth could proceed apparently normally for some considerable time. But some, at least, of these children show a failure to grow which can be detected at the end of the first year of life. This is because, after the nutrition-dependent phase of fetal and infant growth has ended towards the latter part of the first year of life, hGH secretion becomes the predominant controller of the rate of human growth and development.

hGH maintains the normal rate of synthesis of protein in the body, and it also promotes the breakdown of fat for energy use. In its large molecular form, it also has a widespread carbohydrate sparing effect so that it can raise the level of the blood sugar. Thus, a low blood sugar will result in a rise in hGH levels. Its release is also stimulated by stress and trauma through the direct effect of the nervous system on the pituitary gland. hGH has a major influence on increasing the number of cells in the body from late infancy onwards, for it stimulates cell division and DNA formation. Only the brain, and possibly the adrenals and the gonads, are unaffected by it. In particular, hGH is necessary for the proliferation of the cartilage cells of the epiphyseal plates, and so exerts a great effect on height. On the other hand, it has little apparent effect on the maturation of the skeleton.

Although the concentration of hGH in the umbilical cord at birth is higher than in adults, the subsequent daily output does not appear to vary with age, with the stage of puberty, or with the levels of gonadal secretion in the blood. The adolescent spurt does not depend on hGH, but the metabolic effects of the hormone probably continue to be felt throughout adult life, particularly as regards protein synthesis: the amount of hGH in the pituitary appears to remain constant throughout adult life. However, the level in the blood is cyclic over 24 hours, with the highest levels being recorded at night.

Insulin-like growth factors and insulin

hGH operates, at least in part, through the intermediation of secondary growth promoting substances called IGFs or somatomedins. These are peptides which are formed in the liver and other tissues such as bone and fibrous tissue and circulate in the blood plasma. They have several insulin-like effects, which include the stimulation of protein synthesis and the depression of protein breakdown, and indeed it has been said that in any list of growth-promoting peptides insulin itself must come first. (Some Central African pygmies are reported to be deficient in an IGF). There is an age-dependent relationship in scrum levels of the IGFs, with a peak level occurring in adolescence and with a decline in levels after about the age of 50. IGF levels are low in cases of hypopituitism and high in acromegaly.

There is a complicated interaction between hGH and insulin. Insulin and IGFs compete for the same receptor sites and in fact are closely related to one another at the molecular level. There is evidence suggesting that in some cases of diabetes an excess production of hGH may be a factor in depressing insulin production by the islets of Langerhans. There is also an association between the condition of acromegaly and diabetes mellitus.

Children with poor control of their diabetes often suffer from a decrease in their growth velocity while those with a high insulin requirement often are taller and have a delayed puberty. Some evidence suggests that a low level of insulin may in fact stimulate growth.

Growth hormone releasing hormone and somatostatin

The amount of hGH in the bloodstream at a given time is subject to wide variation, following a daily rhythm which varies inversely with the amount of steroid secretion and with the highest levels being recorded during the night. Secretion of hGH is subject to an extremely complex system of checks and counterchecks, feedbacks, and controls. Its release is influenced by the hypothalamus in the brain which produces a growth hormone-releasing hormone (GRF), which is probably secreted in response to a fall in the blood sugar. This hormone is a powerful agent in promoting the release of hGH itself and has been found to be useful in treating children with hGH deficiency.

hGH release is also mediated by somatostatin. This peptide is a growth hormone release-inhibiting factor (SRIF), which not only inhibits hGH release, but also has a direct and powerful inhibiting effect on the receptor sites as well as on other hormones such as gastrin in the stomach and insulin. It is also found in the pancreas, the gut, the brain, and the thyroid gland. There are also claims that the growth of normal animals can be increased by immunosuppression of somatostatin.

As both GRF and SRIF are released by the hypothalamus in the brain, it is not surprising to find that this region of the brain is also influenced by higher centres in the brain, implying a role for the CNS in controlling growth through the effects of the hormones.

The outpouring of hGH is also influenced by such things as the intake of food and the amount of exercise. After injuries, particularly burns, the concentrations of both hGH and IGF-1 in the blood are increased for some time. Like corticosteroids, hGH is secreted intermittently. During sleep, and often during the day as well, bursts of secretion lasting up to 2 hours may occur, and between these bursts the hormone may be impossible to detect in the blood plasma. Secretion during sleep is particularly associated with stage 4 (deep) sleep, and 20–40% of the total 24 hours output occurs in the first 90 minutes of nocturnal sleep. Active secretion appears to take place during only about 6 hours of each day, although lower concentrations of hormone may be found at other times.

Thyroid and parathyroid hormones

The anterior lobe of the pituitary gland also secretes, quite independently, a thyrotrophic hormone, which affects growth by stimulating the thyroid gland to secrete thyroxine and tri-iodothyronine. Both of these stimulate general metabolism, and are particularly important in relation to growth and maturation of the bones, teeth, and brain. The amount of thyroid secretion is thought to decrease somewhat from birth to puberty, at which time there is an interruption of the decline for the period of the adolescent spurt.

If there is a serious deficiency of iodine in the maternal diet, the fetal thyroid may be unable to produce normal amounts of secretion, and the brain fails to develop properly. Similarly, if there is a deficiency of thyroid secretion in childhood, the growth of the whole body suffers, and the child becomes a mentally deficient dwarf. The pituitary and thyroid glands play little direct part in the adolescent spurt, as evidenced by the abrupt changes in the pattern of growth at this time, such as the sudden appearance of the secondary sex characteristics, the closure of the epiphyses, and so on. There may be a relationship with the IGFs as their action on cartilage is affected by the levels of circulating thyroid hormone and low thyroid hormone levels delay growth while high levels are associated with excessive growth.

The parathyroid glands secrete parathormone, which withdraws calcium from the bones to maintain the concentration of calcium in the blood plasma at a constant level. In this it is opposed by another hormone, calcitonin, which is mainly produced by the parafollicular cells of the thyroid gland. Calcitonin inhibits the drain on bone calcium, particularly from bones which are metabolically very active, as they are during growth; it inhibits the action of osteoclasts and increases the numbers of osteoblasts.

Other hormones

There are many other hormones recognized to have effects on growth. Nerve growth factor is related to the IGFs and appears to have a role in the repair of nerves. Epidermal growth factor has a range of actions on cells in the epidermis. Platelet-derived growth factor is released by the platelets when blood clots and may also have a role in cell division. Melatonin, released by the pineal gland, is believed to have a role in regulating puberty as children with pineal tumours often suffer from an unusually early puberty associated with an abnormal pattern of growth. Interestingly, removal of the pineal in chicks seems to result in the development of a spinal curvature (scoliosis), which is itself attributed to a complex growth and nervous system maturation problem. Melatonin also plays a part in the control of the sleep pattern and it has been suggested that this may also be important in the rate of growth.

Steroid hormones and the adrenal glands

The production of hGH and the production of steroids by the adrenal glands appear to oppose each other. Children on long-term corticosteroid therapy for conditions such as asthma suffer an interference with growth, and during such treatment it may be impossible to stimulate growth by administering hGH, even in doses far greater than those necessary to produce a response in children with deficient secretion of the hormone. Recovery of growth can occur when the dosage of corticosteroids is reduced.

Oestrogens stimulate growth at low levels and appear to inhibit growth at high levels. Children with Turner's syndrome can be stimulated to grow if they are given oestrogens.

The glucocorticoids play a part in activating cell division, although high levels are recognized as growth inhibitors.

The appearance of secondary sexual characteristics is attributed to two factors, the first of which is that the cortex of the adrenal glands begins to secrete androgens again. The way in which this happens is not understood; the adrenal cortex is under the control of ACTH produced by the pituitary gland, and has since birth been routinely secreting corticosteroids at a more or less steady level. There is no change in the amount of secretion of ACTH during adolescence, and the other secretions of the adrenal cortex continue steadily on. What, then, causes the cortex to produce an additional secretion? It has been suggested that rising levels of the glucocorticoids during the late fetal period act to suppress adrenal androgen production. Later, stimulation by ACTH overcomes this inhibition and the androgens are activated at the time of puberty. Whatever the mechanism, androgens play a major part in determining the course of the adolescent spurt in both sexes.

The second factor is that just before the adolescent spurt the hypothalamus, which, by producing a gonadotrophin-releasing hormone, has been causing the pituitary to secrete the glycoprotein gonadotrophin throughout childhood, gradually increases its production of the controlling hormone, which is liberated in rhythmic bursts at about 2 hourly intervals during the night. This leads to pulsatile bursts of nocturnal gonadotrophin secretion, which in turn stimulate the interstitial cells of the testicle or ovary to secrete. The gonads of both sexes secrete oestrogens in small quantities from the time of birth onwards. At puberty the oestrogen level rises sharply in girls and to a much more limited extent in boys; the sex difference is possibly due to an inhibitory hormone secreted by the seminiferous tubules of the testicle. Testosterone, produced by the testicle, is important in stimulating growth, as are the androgens, and the steadily rising output of testosterone is responsible for the greater growth of muscles and the greater number of erythrocytes per unit volume in the male. This may be controlled by genes such as *STAT5b* in the male as this gene seems to have a controlling role in muscle development.

The secretions of the ovary have apparently less effect on growth in general, and it follows that in a boy there are two lots of powerful growth-promoting chemicals circulating during the adolescent spurt, while most of the growth in a girl at this time depends on the androgens of the adrenal cortex alone. However, the ovarian secretions largely control the secondary sex changes in the female, including the alterations in the shape of the body. Just how the ovary differentially influences the osteoblasts and osteoclasts of the shoulder and pelvic regions has still to be explained, for there are no obvious differences between the two regions which could account for the effect. Nor is it clear how fat is deposited in certain areas of the body but not in others.

The level of oestrogens in the blood influences the timing of the closure of the epiphyses, and girls who are at risk of becoming excessively tall are sometimes given oestrogens to accelerate the termination of growth. In both sexes it is the androgens which stimulate the development of secondary sexual hair. In the female this is confined to the pubis and the axillae, where the skin is most sensitive to stimulation by androgens, but in the male it extends to adjoining areas of skin and to other regions such as the face, neck, and chest.

Girls of 6–10 years of age mature skeletally much faster than boys, but in girls of 10–15 years the process decelerates relative to boys in the same age group. These stages of maturation are probably endocrine controlled. It seems that the replacement of cartilage by bone is controlled by the thyroid secretion until the time of puberty, but that after puberty the increasing influence of the gonadal hormones overtakes the action of the thyroid, and is responsible for the subsequent maturation patterns of girls and boys. Dental maturity, like skeletal maturity, probably depends on the thyroid gland until the spurt begins, and it is therefore not surprising that dental and skeletal maturity are usually well correlated with each other.

Should there be an excessive production of sex hormones in the growing child, sexual maturation may be considerably advanced. Growth in sexually precocious children usually ceases early, about the age of 10 years, so that they become smaller adults than those with a more normal timetable of development.

Hormonal treatment

Hormonal treatment is now used in an attempt to modify growth if excessive tallness or shortness can be confidently predicted from the bone age and other factors.

To limit height, testosterone can be given to boys and oestrogen to girls. Such treatment precipitates the appearance of the secondary sex characteristics, and hence should not start before the age of about 10. If the radiological age of a girl is over 13 or that of a boy over 14, little success can be expected, but earlier than this some diminution, perhaps 4–5 cm, in the predicted height is possible. The object of treatment is to accelerate skeletal maturation so much that the time left for the child's height to increase is reduced. However, androgens (though not oestrogens) have the drawback that they tend to cause an initial acceleration of growth which may partly nullify the total effect.

Because of the risk of thrombosis inherent in the administration of large doses of oestrogens it is probably not justifiable to use them except in very clear-cut situations. An alternative is to recommend a surgical operation in which the limbs are shortened. There are many ways of achieving this, such as pinning the epiphyses at the lower ends of the femora and the upper ends of the tibiae. As much as 5–10 cm of growth in height may be prevented in this way without causing obvious deformity, because very tall children tend to have somewhat disproportionately long legs.

Surgery can also be used to achieve a considerable lengthening of the femora or tibiae of an excessively small child. Several new techniques have been devised to lengthen bones. In one method, only the cortex of the bone is divided, leaving the medullary cavity intact. Traction is used to pull the pieces apart so that up to 20–30% lengthening can be achieved without unacceptable complications, and without requiring the patient to spend a prolonged period in hospital. Other methods employ traction to the growing epiphysis of the long bone, with often dramatic results. Alternatively the bone is artificially 'fractured' and then reset to achieve a longer bone.

If the child has a deficiency of insulin or thyroid secretion the results of specific replacement of the missing secretion can be remarkable and is of major clinical benefit to the individual. However, hGH itself may not be the panacea for treatment it was once considered to be even when it has seen extensive clinical use in the last decade or so (see Chapter 10). Furthermore, although in the past therapy has used hormones such as androgens in small doses to increase height, there are real risks that exactly the reverse effect may occur if the dose is too large (see above). For the same reasons, the therapeutic use of anabolic steroids has been shown not to increase height beyond what would eventually have been reached without them.

The complexity of the actions of these hormones and growth factors indicates that their role in growth is a complex interaction of control mechanisms and hormonal growth stimulation factors as well as physiological roles which are still not fully understood.

8 Environmental factors influencing growth and maturation

The world we live in affects us all-let's ensure we take great care of it!

Environmental effects on the body

Today we are aware of more and more situations where the growth and maturation of organisms appear to be influenced by events taking place outside their cellular structures. These events can influence the development of the human fetus if they are poisons or infections or even the maternal genetic composition. The growing child can be adversely affected by diet, social environment, or poisons in the atmosphere. Adults and the elderly can be seriously damaged or even killed, for example, by chemicals in the environment or by eating infected food. It is clear that some of these effects may not directly influence growth as such but all have some detrimental effect on the way the body maintains itself in peak condition. Thus we all should appreciate that being green and environmentally aware is important to all and especially to the more vulnerable members of our society.

The word environment is used in the broadest sense so that it includes physical as well as social, cultural, and economic conditions that can affect and influence the growth and development of an individual. Thus the nature of potential environmental threats varies between countries and is frequently linked to economic circumstances. This is a knock-on effect that may lead to health problems, which in turn affect growth. A good example is a lack of an adequate water supply associated with poor drains and sanitation which may result in high levels of water-borne disease leading in turn to a grossly magnified effect on the growing individual.

Thus the environment a child grows up in can have a marked effect on its physical development.

Public health is a critical factor in understanding these effects and highlighting new ones. Potential new threats now have arisen from the very technologies which have enabled us to exploit and control our environment very successfully, as we are now potentially overloading the capacity of the world to absorb waste and pollution, frequently on a transnational basis. The effects of the nuclear accident in the reactor at Chernobyl were felt in many countries and we still do not know the full effects this accident is likely to have on the growth and development of individuals potentially affected. Environmental pollution from chemicals is also known to affect individuals and their growth and clearly poses a risk to the unborn child. Pesticides and agricultural fertilizers are also widely dispersed in the environment and can find their way into the food chain, with impacts on health found retrospectively. Although little is really known about the relationship between chemical release or use and their interaction with growing individuals, we are aware that there is a dose-related response which varies with age, so that the youngest child is likely to be more vulnerable than an adult. It is an area where the lack of scientific knowledge of effects leaves us uncertain whether there is a risk to growth.

Nutrition

An adequate supply of food is essential for individuals to achieve a normal growth pattern and maximize their potential as adults. The intake of food supplies a growing child with its nutritional requirements and there are many studies which have shown the close relationship between this supply and growth. The evidence for this received considerable support in analysis of data collected during the 1914–18 and 1939–45 wars where famines which occurred during the hostilities retarded the growth of many children. For example, in the Netherlands, the winter famine of 1944–45 severely impaired children's growth. In post-war Germany, under similar near famine conditions, children lagged 10–20 months behind normal growth performance, and in Japan the mean height of adults fell between 1945 and 1949 and only returned its previous levels in 1956.

It has also been observed that the recovery in growth rate after periods of famine occurs faster in cities than in rural areas, suggesting that individuals in these environments may have better nutritional intakes than rural inhabitants.

Human malnutrition involves not only a deficiency of calories, but a lack of specific foodstuffs, and it is impossible to separate the two factors. Several experiments on supplementation of inadequate diets have been carried out under conditions of widespread malnutrition and famine and these have shown that the preadolescent growth period is most severely affected. There are ethical problems involved in studies in this field so most of our knowledge on the relation of nutrition to growth derives from animal work.

When rats and mice are fed on a diet deficient in calories but otherwise satisfactory, they cease to grow but can resume growth when an adequate supply of calories is restored. Rats have been kept immature for up to 1000 days on such a diet, and were still juvenile while their fellows on a normal diet were senile. On starting normal feeding, the rats rapidly grew to adult size, although those which had been kept on the deficient diet for more than 3 years could not always begin growing again. Subsequent work showed that the diet which results in the maximal final size of experimental animals is one which, as judged by appetite and by growth rate, represents a moderate degree of caloric under-feeding.

The human need for calories varies with the phase of development. In the first year of life a baby requires about twice as many calories per unit weight as a male adult doing moderately heavy work, and a schoolboy going through his adolescent spurt may require as much as 3000 kcal a day. He also needs about 50% more calcium, nitrogen, and vitamin D than he did before the spurt began.

Nutrition also affects the rate of maturity. Malnourished children exhibit delayed growth and also a delayed puberty. Body proportions at birth such as weight related to length are also a good indicator of a time of restraint of growth during pregnancy. After a period of human or animal malnutrition has ended, growth accelerates in an attempt to compensate for the loss in height and weight. This 'catch-up growth' can be successful in restoring normality if the period of malnutrition has been short. Sometimes complete compensation proves impossible as, even if puberty is delayed, the longer growth period available cannot compensate for the lost growth in preadolescence due to the dietary deficiencies. The phenomenon of catch-up growth raises interesting questions regarding the central control of growth, and the capacity of the body to return to a genetically determined growth curve after having been pushed off it has been termed 'homoeorrhesis'. Furthermore, evidence suggests that restraints on the growth of a fetus resulting in small size at birth or poor nutrition in infancy may influence the incidence of cardiovascular and other diseases in later life (see Box 8.1)

Undernutrition tends to produce differential growth. For example, the growth of the teeth takes precedence over the growth of the bones, and the bones grow better than the soft tissues, such as muscle and fat. Skeletal maturation is retarded less than skeletal growth, and myelination in the brain is less affected than total brain growth. The growth of the sexual organs at puberty is relatively less depressed than that of other tissues and organs. Restriction of food slows down production in the germinative layer of the skin, but also decreases the rate of loss from the surface, so that the thickness of the skin remains relatively normal.

Milk has also a powerful influence on growth. Studies undertaken in Scotland in 1928 showed that supplementation of the diet with extra milk produced faster growth. This is probably due to the extra proteins in milk. Peoples who normally have a diet rich in milk, such as the Turkana in Kenya, East Africa, are generally taller.

Box 8.1

Recent studies have shown that it is possible that the nutrition of the fetus and new-born child may have a significant effect on the health of the adult. David Barker and colleagues in Southampton discovered the existence of unique medical records of babies born in Hertfordshire dating from the 1920s which allowed the research team to trace and follow up the same individuals as adults. If the subjects had died, the cause of death was sought out. The findings were able to link poor nutrition and poor health of the mother and baby to the onset in later life of medical conditions, such as high blood pressure, heart disease, respiratory disease and diabetes. The studies suggest that not only is growth affected by nutritional influences during the early and later growing years but that adult health is as well. Small size at birth or reduced early growth appears to be causally linked to cardiovascular disease in later life. The findings indicate that improvements in the health and nutrition of expectant mothers is an important contribution not only to the growth potential of their children but is also important in preventing chronic ill health in later life.

The role of proteins

Starvation or semi-starvation also alters the composition of the body. Protein is not only not added to, but is used up, so that the cell mass of the body is reduced. Fat is also used up, but the extracellular body fluid is actually increased. The loss of weight may thus be partly masked by what is known as famine oedema. The mechanism whereby this increase in body water occurs is not yet clearly understood.

As regards the detailed composition of a diet suitable for normal growth, much remains to be discovered. There must be an adequate supply of protein, which is the most important single item: nine different amino acids have been claimed to be essential for growth, and absence of any one will result in disordered or stunted growth. Protein malnutrition is a major factor in the condition known as kwashiorkor, in which there is a general slowing down of skeletal growth and maturation; the delay in epiphyseal fusion may be as much as a year compared with normally nourished children, and puberty may be delayed. The muscles shrink, there is considerable subcutaneous oedema, and fats accumulate in the liver.

On the other hand, marasmus, which occurs more in younger children than does kwashiorkor, is due to a deficiency of both protein and carbohydrate. There is no oedema, and there is gross wasting of muscles. In dealing with famine victims it is important to assess the body mass index (BMI). In adults a BMI of 18–20 indicates mild starvation, one of 16–18 moderate starvation, and a figure below 16 severe starvation necessitating hospital treatment. In children between the ages of 1 and 5 years, a measurement of the circumference of the mid-point of the arm is used: about 16 cm is normal for this age group; 13.5 cm is taken as the threshold of starvation; and a measurement below 12.5 cm indicates a serious problem.

Trace elements

Other factors such as trace elements are also essential for growth. Zinc plays a part in protein synthesis and is a constituent of certain enzymes. A deficiency of zinc causes stunting, interference with sexual development, and falling out of hair, and it has been suggested that intracellular zinc deficiency may be a cause of senescence.

Iodine is needed for the manufacture of thyroid hormones. Bone will not grow properly without an adequate supply of calcium, phosphorus, and other inorganic constituents such as magnesium. Manganese is needed to ensure the development of cartilage and its deficiency could well affect the development of the bones and joints.

In growing children, about 180 mg of calcium is added to the bones each day, rising to 400 mg at the height of the adolescent spurt. Fluorine has been shown to harden tooth enamel and to protect against decay and it also plays a part in bone formation.

Iron is required for the production of haemoglobin, and a deficiency of iron is probably the commonest nutritional deficiency in the world. The average loss of blood in menstruation contains about 0.5 mg of iron a day, and it follows that women need more iron in their diet than men. Yet their intake is often considerably less, specially if they are on a weight-reducing diet, and the result is iron-deficiency anaemia. This is common in adolescent girls who have begun menstruating, are still growing, and are often restricting their food intake.

Infestation by parasites such as hookworm interferes with growth by causing a loss of blood and protein from the intestinal wall: there is evidence that some parasites such as tapeworms may also interfere with absorption of foodstuffs. In view of the world-wide distribution of the helminths, this is an important problem.

Vitamins

Vitamin A is thought to control the activities of both osteoblasts and osteoclasts. Too much vitamin A in the diet, which may occur when people take large amounts of vitamin preparations unnecessarily, can cause skeletal growth to slow down. On the other hand, a lack of vitamin A causes defects in the moulding process at the ends of the bones, so that clumsily thickened bones result, and the nerve trunks which run through holes in the skull may be pressed upon because the holes do not enlarge with growth as they should do.

Vitamin B_2 has a considerable general influence on growth, which is severely impaired in deficiency.

In vitamin C deficiency the intercellular substance of bone is inadequately formed, and newly constructed cartilage lacks collagen. Gross deficiency causes scurvy, a disease in which, among other things, there is a decreased growth rate at the epiphyseal plates, and deficient bone formation there and elsewhere, so that both the region of the plates and the shafts of the bones are easily broken. Calcification is not interfered with.

In contrast, vitamin D deficiency is the cause of rickets, in which there is distorted growth in the region of the epiphyseal plates, as a result of deficient calcification of the cartilage there. This is because vitamin D stimulates the absorption of calcium from the intestine and possibly also the reabsorption of calcium by the kidney tubules. If there is too little vitamin D, there is therefore an inadequate supply of calcium and phosphorus in the bloodstream, and in gross cases the softened bones may become distorted and bent under the weight of the body (Fig. 8.1). Rickets is once again a significant disease in certain places in Britain, where the adolescent diet may be deficient in both vitamin D and calcium and where the children are unable to synthesize adequate amounts of vitamin D in their skin because of the lack of sunlight.

The active derivative of vitamin D which is produced in the body has been found to assist in controlling cell division and differentiation in malignant tumours, and it has been suggested that it may regulate cellular metabolism by altering intracellular calcium concentrations.

Altitude

The effect of altitude on growth has been extensively studied. Children brought up at high altitudes tend to grow more slowly and may be smaller than those living at lower levels. Children living in Colorado in the USA often exhibit prenatal growth retardation and this can continue into later childhood and adolescence. The effect is that adult height attained is reduced. Similar effects occur in children living at high altitude in South America. The causes of this slowing of growth are likely to be the effect of a low oxygen pressure in the atmosphere, which leads to less oxygen getting into the body. This effect is called hypoxia. The body copes with the hypoxia by creating more red blood cells which carry more blood from the lungs to the growing tissues, but this appears unable to fully counter the effects due to the lower oxygen pressure.

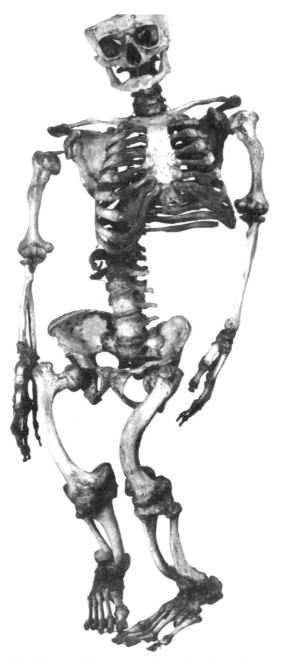

Fig. 8.1 Rickets. The skeleton of 'bowed Joseph', who led the Meal Riots in Edinburgh, and died in 1780. Notice the gross distortion of the bones of the lower limb and the spine, and the shortening of the arms. Probably other factors as well as rickets were partly responsible for the condition. (Photograph by kind permission of Professor G. J. Romanes, Department of Anatomy, Edinburgh University.)

Oxygen

Problems with the circulation of blood in the baby and young child can affect the growth rate. Children born with a congenital cardiac defect, of whatever sort, may, if the disturbance is severe enough, show a stunting and retardation of growth. If the defect can be corrected by surgical repair, normal growth may result. The cause of the interference with growth is not clear; it is not simply due to the tissues receiving too little oxygen for normal metabolism, for the severity of the defect and the amount of interference with growth do not always run parallel. Furthermore, congenital cardiac defects which do not lead to deficient oxygenation of the blood may also be accompanied by impairment of growth.

The delay in growth which occurs in some severe cases of asthma is, however, associated with marked obstruction of the flow of air.

Secular trends

There are impressive series of figures which show that children nowadays are growing faster than formerly. The average height of recruits to the Norwegian Army in 1875 was 1.3 cm more than it was in 1825 in recruits of the same age; by 1935 the average was over 5 cm more than in 1825. Similar, and perhaps more homogeneous, figures from Marlborough College in England showed that the average height of 16-year-old boys increased by more than 1.3 cm every 10 years from 1873 to 1943.

A similar trend was found in younger children. Between 1880 and 1950 the average height of American and west European children between the ages of 5 and 7 years increased by more than 1.3 cm every 10 years for a total of more than 10 cm. German, Polish, and Danish figures all confirmed the general result, and interestingly enough the increase was not confined to the less well-off children. It follows that the phenomenon was probably not simply due to better nutrition in terms of calories, for one would expect an improvement due to this cause to be more marked in the poorer people than in the wealthy, who would presumably have been eating well all the time. It is possible that the balance rather than the quantity of the diet may have been a factor. Since 1950 the trend has at last flattened off in the developed countries such as the United States and Britain. This is attributed to the fact that the children of the affluent in Western Europe and America are now receiving a diet which is maximally efficient in promoting growth. The secular difference in height in adults is not nearly so marked as in children: adults are probably getting larger, but much more slowly than children of a given age. Cross-sectional data may be very misleading, and longitudinal data are as yet too scarce to enable any firm pronouncement to be made.

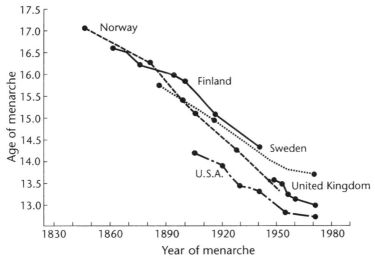

Fig. 8.2 Secular trends in the age of menarche, 1845–1960. The graphs are based largely on interrogation of schoolchildren and young adults, but some of the early figures depend on the memories of older people. (From Tanner, J. M. (1962). *Growth at adolescence* (2nd edn). Blackwell Scientific Publications, Oxford, by kind permission of the author and publishers.)

In Britain weight has increased secularly more than height, so that the adult male population (at least) has become progressively heavier at a given age. Between 1850 and 1950 the average increase in weight of adolescents was about 2.3 kg per decade, and the most recent figures show that young and middle-aged men today are about 7 kg heavier than men of similar age and height 30 years ago. In earlier studies the incidence of obesity increased with age until at least 55 years, but it appears that it now increases until about 35, after which it flattens off.

One of the most striking of the features which indicated a secular trend in maturation corresponding to the secular trends in growth was a progressive advancement in the timing of the menarche (Fig. 8.2). The figures for this trend could not be extrapolated backwards as they would have indicated that in the Middle Ages people never menstruated until late in life, whereas the historical evidence available suggests that puberty occurred about the age of 14 in medieval Europe as opposed to about 13 nowadays. The extrapolation of the curve forwards was equally alarming, as it indicated that in a few years' time girls might be menstruating as babies. This was also an improbable inference, and in fact the advancement of the menarche, like the trend to increased size, levelled off after 1950 in Britain, north-west Europe, and the United States. Elsewhere in Europe it appears to have continued, although more slowly. It has been suggested that the observations in Fig. 8.2 represent a recovery from a significant retardation of the menarche during the time of the industrial revolution. If this is true, the problem is to explain the cause of the hypothetical retardation. The revolution itself cannot have been an all-important factor, as figures from Scandinavia, where the revolution occurred much later and was much less violent, show an exactly similar trend. A more probable reason for the advancement of the menarche is the progressive increase in the adequacy of nutrition in Europe and elsewhere. Nevertheless, the same reservations must be made in respect of this theory as were made in relation to the secular changes in height and weight.

If epiphyseal fusion results from the secretion of hormones activated at puberty, it follows that the earlier puberty occurs the sooner the individual stops growing, and this might lead one to expect a secular decrease, rather than an increase, in the height of adults. The explanation of why this has not occurred probably lies in the fact that the children in whom the earlier puberty occurs are already taller than their predecessors, and this factor outweighs the earlier cessation of growth.

A small secular improvement in the intelligence quotient (IQ) has been reported from several developed countries, but the interpretation to be placed on this is obscure; it may simply mean that children (and teachers) have become more familiar with the sort of questions asked in intelligence tests. The evidence suggests that there is an increasing superiority of girls over boys as regards IQ at the age of 11 years, and this has been related to evidence indicating that the adolescent spurt in physical growth is occurring earlier.

Socio-economic class

Studies of the effect of socio-economic conditions on growth have a very long history both in the medical field as well as in the fields of psychology and sociology. There is a considerable body of evidence which shows that differences in the standard of living have more effect on growth in height than anything else, with children in the top socio-economic groups being taller than the children of unskilled labourers. In Britain, this class difference can be as much as 2.5 cm at 3 years of age and about 4.5 cm at adolescence. Not only do we find that such children forming the higher socio-economic groups are taller, but their rate of growth is faster and they tend to become taller adults. This effect has been shown to mirror closely the fathers' and mothers' educational achievement, especially in developing countries. Unfortunately, in many European countries, especially the United Kingdom, the gap between the rich and poor is widening, so the inequality in health, as mirrored by life expectancies and disease incidences, also widens and the growth potential of the different classes of children is consequently affected. Clearly this raises a considerable number of problems in the field of both growth and development where there is a considerable body of evidence to support a relationship between income and life expectancy.

Where we examine the difference in weight, the effect is less marked, but in the same direction. Many European and North American studies show the individuals in lower social classes are smaller and have more body fat. In the USA, poorer leaner girls grow up to be fatter women when compared with better off women. They then have babies of a lower birth weight, and these babies tend to grow up smaller and heavier in turn. Furthermore, the same group also seem to underachieve in education and may have a lower IQ. Such differences have become obliterated in Sweden where social class distinctions have become blurred.

The findings suggest that lower social class effects are cumulative and not due to prenatal and infantile influences alone.

Another problem which is now becoming a major contributing factor to poorer socio-economic conditions is that of the single parent family. We know that single or lone parents headed about 23% of all families in Britain in 1994 and the vast majority of these are headed by women. What is not yet clear is the change society will have on the children of single parent families but, based on evidence from other sources, it is quite likely that these children will be at risk of poor nutrition which will be reflected in their not growing as well as the better off and consequently they will be more likely to suffer from ill-health in later life.

Family conflict and disturbances to the family unit such as divorce, separation, or desertion by parents is also thought to affect growth, suggesting that stress may affect the amount of growth hormone produced. A recent study undertaken in London showed that children from these backgrounds were more than twice as likely to be below average height. Such scientific evidence indicates how the environment one grows up in can serve to have life-long consequences.

However, socio-economic differences are not simply a matter of food, and probably several causes are involved. The economic factor seems to be less important than the provision of a home where meals are regular, adequate, and balanced, where sleep and exercise are sufficient, and where the children are taught the basic rules of health. The Carnegie Task Force concluded that factors such as full-term birth, normal birth-weight, growing up in a family with two dependable adults, and living in a supportive and safe community are important positive factors contributing to the best environment for growth. The size of the family also appears to be important, for children in large families are usually smaller and lighter, and have less chance of becoming obese, than children in small families. Possibly this is because in large families children tend to get less individual care and attention.

The role of urbanization has also been examined in many studies. Work has always attracted people to the larger towns and cities and consequently, the better economic status of the employed has resulted in children growing up better fed, healthier and taller than children from similar backgrounds in rural communities. Such children also mature earlier. However, sweeping generalizations in this context are risky as the poor living in slum dwellings in the Third World are smaller due to the economic effects of an inability to provide a good diet resulting in poor nutrition.

The complications of pregnancy have also been found to exert an influence on the growth of the child. Severe complications of pregnancy, labour, and birth affect the physical development of the children of lower socio-economic status families far more that those from the better off.

These factors, together with the others considered in this chapter, emphasize the caution with which growth charts must be approached; charts and curves derived from children of a high social class in an economically advanced country may well be quite different from those taken from children of a lower class in an economically backward country.

Disease

We have already indicated that poor socio-economic conditions can lead to ill-health in the child with the consequential effect this has on their growth. The Black report of 1980 showed that inequalities in health persist in the twentieth century in Britain and that, in spite of provision of a good health service, the social inequalities in society are reflected in the health of the population. Children from poorer families are more likely to have more illnesses than the better-off and there is evidence of a gradient of increased mortality associated with increasing disadvantage, most marked at ages 1–4 years. Boys appear more at risk than girls. Furthermore, in spite of a steep decline in infant mortality, the gap between classes still remains depressingly large. OECD (Organization for Economic Cooperation and Development) figures reveal a direct relationship between the percentage of the population in relative poverty and the infant mortality rate and we also know that accident rates are much higher for children from these lower groups.

Disregarding the influence of social class, disease in childhood has an impact which is similar to that of malnutrition with good examples afforded by tuberculosis, kidney disease, cerebral palsy, and cystic fibrosis. Asthma may lead to a delay in puberty, but final height is within normal expectations.

Many drugs have either positive or negative effects on appetite, absorption, and metabolism, and drugs which stimulate excretion, such as purgatives and diuretics, may have an important effect in lowering the necessary body content of minerals such as potassium.

The best known example of a drug which has a deleterious effect on growth is that due to long-term steroid therapy. Treatment with glucocorticoids slows growth and also leads to progressive loss of bone, particularly trabecular bone. After disease or drug therapy ends there is an acceleration comparable with that following the end of a time of malnutrition, and again this homoeorrhesis may or may not completely compensate for the loss of growth during the period of illness. Girls seem to be more resistant to the effects of outside influences interfering with growth than boys, and after the influence has ceased to operate they 'catch up' with their normal curve more rapidly.

Maturation times in the female are also less affected by extraneous factors such as health and environment. In both sexes there is a homoeorrhetic spurt in maturation following illness, and this keeps pace with the spurt in growth.

If piglets are delivered by Caesarean section under aseptic conditions, and reared with minimal opportunities of acquiring any infectious disease, they mature faster; it is probable that similar considerations apply to humans.

Just how general diseases cause slowing of growth is not known, but an obvious factor is reduced food intake caused by poor appetite. There may also be a diminution in the secretion of growth hormone, resulting from an increase in the secretion of corticosteroids from the adrenal cortex. There is a decrease in the mitotic index of the cartilage cells in the epiphyseal plates, and this, for a time at least, is not accompanied by a decrease in the rate of ossification. The epiphyseal plates therefore become thinner, and the number of cells available to produce more cartilage becomes reduced.

Antenatal insults

Children born to alcoholic mothers may have facial and other abnormalities characteristic of the 'fetal alcoholic syndrome'.

Subsequent growth and development are retarded, and in a recent Scottish investigation 'catch-up' growth did not occur. It is possible that lesser intakes of alcohol during pregnancy may also retard the growth of the child.

Consumption of alcohol is often associated with consumption of tobacco, and there is some evidence that smoking by the mother during pregnancy, which is already known to cause a lower birth weight and an increased mortality at about the time of birth, can also influence later growth and development. In a large-scale controlled investigation the 7-year-old children of mothers who had smoked more than 10 cigarettes a day during pregnancy were on the average 1 cm shorter and 3–5 months retarded in reading ability when compared with children of non-smoking mothers. Further analysis of the same group of children indicates the probability that these deficiencies may persist into adult life, the evidence being stronger in relation to intellectual development than to height.

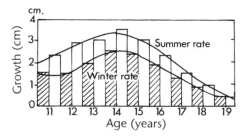

Fig. 8.3 Effects of season on growth. Half-yearly increments of growth in German cadets, 1902; growth in the summer months is more rapid than in the winter. Notice that the difference between summer and winter is greatest about the time of adolescent spurt, and becomes less noticeable as maturity is neared. (From Thompson, D'Arcy W. (1942). *Growth and form* (2nd edn). Cambridge University Press, London, by kind permission of the publishers.)

Undernutrition at the critical period of maximum growth velocity can cause permanent stunting of experimental animals, and this is associated with a deficiency in the numbers of cells in the organs of the animals. Similarly 'small for dates' full-term babies whose intrauterine growth was slow are likely to continue to grow and develop slowly after birth.

Seasonal effects

There is a large amount of evidence which suggests that growth in height is faster in the spring and summer than in the autumn by a factor of $2-2\frac{1}{2}$ times (Fig. 8.3). On the contrary, growth in weight proceeds faster (sometimes four or five times faster) in the autumn than in the spring. Children thus tend to grow in height in the early part of the year and to fill out in the latter part, although individuals may show a rhythm different from that of the majority.

In the Gambia, subsistence farming communities have a good food supply during the dry months and children show faster growth rates associated with the good food supply. In the rainy season, the decline in quality of the food supply is mirrored by a slower growth rate in the children.

In addition to the food supply effects associated with seasonality, there are undoubtedly other reasons why a seasonal difference in growth exists. One of these may be related to sunlight exposure. Although the amount of daylight exposure may be important, as it is a potent stimulus in other ways in the animal world, studies involving totally blind children are inconclusive since their fastest and slowest growth periods may occur in any season. The case in favour of sunlight playing a part in growth is supported by the fact that humans synthesize vitamin D3 in the skin and this vitamin is essential for bone growth.

The seasonal tides of growth make it essential to measure any patient suspected of a growth disturbance over a full year, for in autumn and winter growth in the height of children between the ages of 5 and 9 years may be less than the measurement error.

At other ages the seasonal variations may be outweighed by overall changes of much greater magnitude.

Perhaps the most startling example of seasonal growth in animals is provided by the antlers of deer, in which every tissue concerned grows at a rate much in excess of its normal potential. Thus, the branches of the trigeminal nerve supplying the antlers may grow at a rate of as much as 12 mm a day.

Climate

There are suggestions that climate plays a part in growth, although the evidence is doubtful as it is difficult to separate these effects from racial, dietary, and other effects such as those produced by disease.

However, each major race of humankind varies in stature according to the climate in which it lives. Thus, a colder climate is inhabited by people who are heavier, with a larger trunk and shorter legs such as in Scandinavia and northern Europe generally. In contrast, people living in hot climates have lighter trunks and longer legs, such as exhibited by Africans. This is due to the need to get rid of excess heat acquired from the environment and this is achieved by having a large body area from which evaporation and radiation can take place. In the colder climates, the smaller surface area of the larger trunk and shorter limbs reduces this heat loss.

Interestingly, races living in the tropical rain-forests have adapted to the high humidity by evolving a small body size which reduces heat loss by evaporation but maximizes the loss achieved by radiation and conduction. Both African Pygmies and Amazonian Indians are examples of this adaption.

Exercise

It has already been mentioned that adults can increase the size of their muscles by exercise. The same holds good in children, although when the body is growing longitudinally the result is less marked than it is later, when the epiphyses have closed. As in adults, there appears to be no increase in the number of muscle fibres,

Surprisingly, an Australian study has shown that male and female children aged 10 or 11 years who had been subjected to intensive strength and flexibility training for 2 years as 'State-level' swimmers did not differ from matched controls in height, weight, strength, or flexibility, although they were superior in cardiovascular fitness.

Exercise is capable of reducing the storage depots of fat, and by so doing may alter the shape of the body and its composition. Inactivity is an important cause of obesity in children.

Emotion

A well-known experiment in post-war Germany showed the importance of emotional factors in growth. Two similar orphanages were selected for a dietary experiment. After a control period during which both institutions had the same diet, the children in the first orphanage were given a supplement to their diet. To the surprise of the experimenter, the growth of the children given the supplement actually fell behind that of the children in the other orphanage who were given no supplement. Investigation showed that the result was due to the transfer, at the same time as the control period ended, of an unpleasant superintendent from the second orphanage to the first. This female martinet used to take the children to task at the time when they were eating, and the severe strain imposed in this manner apparently outweighed the importance of the dietary supplement. The matter was clinched when it was found that she had transferred with her some of her 'favourites' from the second orphanage: these children had thrived under the original conditions, and grew even faster when given the supplement to the diet.

Emotional disturbances are a not uncommon cause of failure to grow normally, and the victims often show a bizarre and sometimes excessive appetite. They have been described as 'trash-can raiders'.

It is not known how emotion influences growth, but there are several possibilities. It may be that it affects the supposed hypothalamic growth centre, or that it disturbs metabolism, or that increased amounts of steroids are produced. There may be associated dietary deficiencies in domestic cases of 'psychosocial dwarfism'. It has been suggested that such children may not get enough stage 4 sleep; if so, the growth hormone production might be diminished. However, treatment with growth hormone has not proved successful.

9   Growth and repair

What wound did ever heal but by degrees?
Shakespeare

Growth cycles: wear and tear

The external environment exerts a major influence on all parts of the body due to it causing repeated minor damage, injury, and other effects. This requires growth process mechanisms by the body to ensure effective continuous replacement, a process which is not restricted solely to childhood and the growing period, but one which continues throughout the whole of adult life.

The most obvious example of this process affects the skin and its appendages. Here, the superficial layer of the epidermis is constantly worn away and shed, but the epidermis as a whole is maintained at a constant thickness by the continual growth of the stem cells lying in the deepest layer which replace the loss. The daughter cells produced by this germinative layer (Fig. 9.1) are gradually pushed towards the surface by the steady division of the stem cells, and arrive there after about 15–20 days in the case of the forearm skin: the time varies somewhat in other regions. During this journey the cells lose their nuclei and their cytoplasm is progressively converted into keratin, a protein which serves to protect the deeper layers. The production and differentiation of these keratinocytes is under the control of chemical factors released from the fibroblasts of the dermis. In the common skin disease called psoriasis something goes wrong with this mechanism; stem cells are increased in number and there is a great rise in the number of mitotic figures in the epidermis. The production of new cells is thus enormously increased: in a square centimetre of skin some 1250 cells a day are produced in a normal person, but in psoriasis about 35 000 are manufactured.

Activity in the germinative layer of the epidermis can be detected by the appearance of mitotic figures. As might be expected, the skin does not grow all over the body at a constant rate, and regions which are subject to much friction exhibit more mitotic figures than regions which are more protected. There is also a diurnal rhythm of activity; for example, the cells in the prepuce of an infant show more figures between the hours of 9 p.m. and 10 p.m. than between 5 a.m and 10 a.m. In animals as well as humans the mitotic rate is high during rest or sleep periods, and low during wakefulness or activity. This has

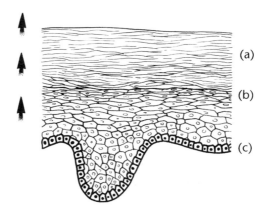

Fig. 9.1 Growth of epidermis. (a) Layer of stem cells (germinative layer) in the depths of the epidermis. (b) As the cells produced by the germinative layer are pushed towards the surface (and so further from their blood supply), they become flattened, lose their nuclei and die. (c) The remains of the cells lose their identity and become converted into layers of keratin (cornified layer). Ultimately flakes of keratin are lost from the surface of the skin by attrition.

been correlated with the levels of adrenaline and corticosteroids in the blood, which are high during activity and low during rest. It has been suggested that all diurnal rhythms of this kind are in part controlled by the circulating 'stress' hormones of the adrenal, which are supposed to interact with the local growth regulating mechanisms to suppress mitosis.

The growth of the skin adjusts itself to the varying surface area of the adult body. If there is a rapid and considerable gain in weight, the skin grows to cover the increased volume. Sometimes the volume may increase so rapidly that the skin cannot keep pace; for example, in pregnancy some areas of skin on the abdominal wall may become stretched and thinned, so giving rise to the characteristic shiny patches known as striae gravidarum.

When weight is lost in adult life, the elasticity of the skin adjusts it to the lessened surface area, and skin growth becomes correspondingly depressed to keep pace with the needs of the body. If the loss of weight occurs after the elastic fibres have degenerated in old age, the stretched skin hangs in loose wrinkles over the reduced body surface.

The cycle of growth, degeneration, loss, and repair characteristic of normal skin applies also to the hairs covering the body, which are constantly shed and replaced. The long hairs of the scalp have a life of several years, and the shorter hairs of the body may last for a year or so; the cycle is thus a much longer one than that of the epidermal cells. In all cases hairs tend to be replaced by other hairs, although in later life replacement is not complete. The root of the old hair is absorbed in a manner which is not completely understood, and the detached hair shaft is pushed towards the surface by the

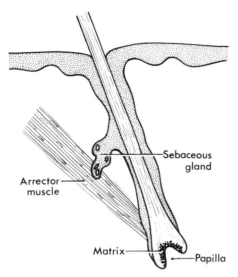

Fig. 9.2 Growth of hair. The cells of the matrix surrounding the papilla of the hair divide continually, so adding to the length of the hair and forcing it up its tubular follicle.

activity of the cells forming the sheath of the hair, until eventually it falls out. A new hair is then produced by the division of cells in the 'matrix' of the follicle (Fig. 9.2), and grows up the follicle until it reaches the surface.

In every hair the period of growth is followed by a quiescent phase which ends in death. In the rat, all the body hairs show the same total life cycle of about 35 days, half being growth and half quiescence.

Because hair replacement occurs in 'waves', it is relatively simple to determine the lifetime of rat hairs. In humans, replacement occurs in scattered groups, so that some hairs in a small area of skin may be actively growing, while others are inactive or dying. In consequence, it is not easy to tell whether there is a standard life cycle which applies to every hair.

The rate of growth varies with the texture of the hair: coarse hair grows faster than fine hair. Hair grows more rapidly in summer than in winter, but it is unaffected by repeated cutting, or by exposure to sunshine. Every day between 20 and 75 scalp hairs are moulted, and the scalp hair grows at the rate of about 2.1 mm a week; the corresponding rate for the beard is higher, perhaps 2.8 mm. The hair on the legs of children grows at a rate of 1.4 mm a week; this increases to nearly 2 mm a week by the age of 40–45 years.

The axillary hairs grow 2.2 mm a week, and this rate is unaffected by age. Hair may continue to grow at its normal rate even though other tissues in the body are severely retarded by malnutrition.

There is a hereditary tendency towards the development of baldness in males, and it is interesting that castration appears to keep this in check. The administration of male sex hormone does not in itself produce baldness, but if it is given to castrates it will permit the genetic factor to operate, so that the individual will become bald. It is well known that hereditary baldness is very unusual in women.

The growth of nails differs in some respects from that of the hairs. In the first place, it is slowed by old age, poor nutrition, and infectious diseases. Secondly, damage to the nails, such as is produced by nail biting, leads to 20% higher rate of growth.

The finger-nails grow about four times as fast as the toe-nails, and this effect is not yet explained, although a contributory factor may be that the finger-nails are trimmed more frequently than the toe-nails. The average growth of the thumb-nail is about 4 cm a year, and the rate appears to depend in part on the amount of usage, for when the hand is immobilized because of injury the growth of the nails is considerably slowed. This may be the reason why nail growth in the non-dominant hand is slower. Like the hairs, the nails grow faster in the summer than in the winter.

Less is known about the repair and replacement of other surface structures. The epithelia of the respiratory and urinary apparatus renew themselves comparatively slowly, but those of the intestinal tract are renewed very rapidly. In this instance, the new cells are formed in the crypts of the intestine and migrate along the villi to their tips, from which they are shed into the lumen of the gut. In the rat, the mucosa of the small intestine is completely replaced every 34 hours, and it is probable that the cycle is of similar length in humans; mitotic figures are very common in the human intestine. It has been calculated that a rat loses daily about one-twentieth of the total cell population of its whole body.

In vitamin A deficiency, certain epithelial surfaces fail to shed their dead cells and in consequence become dry and thickened. The cornea may soften and ultimately disintegrate, causing blindness.

The source of the injury responsible for cyclical death and replacement is not necessarily an external one. The circulating erythrocytes have to squeeze through narrow channels during the whole of their life in the vascular system, and they have no nucleus which might enable them to undertake 'running repairs'. As a result they become worn out after a life of approximately 120 days, and their condition is in some way recognized by the cells of the reticuloendothelial system, which seize and destroy them. The loss is made good by the stem cells of the red bone marrow in the vertebrae, the flat bones, and the ends of the long bones; a deficit of half a litre or so of blood can be fully restored in the course of a few days. After repeated haemorrhages, red marrow is found in the shafts of the long bones, indicating the immense effort the body has been making to replace the loss. If the marrow fails to keep up a balancing supply of new cells, the erythrocyte count falls and the patient becomes anaemic.

Growth activity in the reproductive tract

The genital apparatus in both male and female affords examples of continual growth activity. In the testicle the spermatozoa are produced by stem cells in the walls of the seminiferous tubules, and are gradually pushed out of the testicle by the pressure of their fellows. It is not known how long they live in the tubes of the male genital system, but each ejaculation contains up to 100 million spermatozoa, and their life outside the body is very short. In animals, spermatogenesis takes place in 'waves' of activity which pass along the seminiferous tubules.

The ovary has a fairly regular cycle of growth which results in the production of one mature ovum (rarely two) every month or so. There is considerable variation in the exact timing, which may indeed differ in the same woman from cycle to cycle. Most women have a cyclical period of between 25 and 35 days, and a 28-day cycle is accepted as the average. One (or possibly two) of the primary oocytes present in the ovary at puberty becomes coated by a layer of cells which divide and eventually surround a cavity (Fig. 9.3). During this time the primary oocyte undergoes the first stage of a reduction division which forms a secondary oocyte plus a polar body containing the excess and discarded chromosomal material. Further growth in size of the whole apparatus, which is now known as a Graafian follicle, is followed by bursting of the follicle, so allowing the mature secondary oocyte and its covering membranes and cell layers to be shed into the uterine tube. If fertilization by a spermatozoon takes place within the tube, the second stage of division occurs which results in the formation of the mature ovum and a second polar body.

The cavity from which the secondary oocyte was expelled becomes filled with a blood clot, and the cells of its walls multiply to form a yellow structure called the corpus luteum. If pregnancy does not supervene, this becomes converted into scar tissue, forming a corpus albicans. However, if the ovum is fertilized, it embeds itself in the wall of the uterus and this reprieves the corpus luteum of menstruation, which grows and becomes the corpus luteum of pregnancy, an endocrine gland which secretes hormones until about the fifth or sixth month of pregnancy.

Corresponding with and influenced by the ovarian cycles are the cycles of growth, death, and shedding of the inner layers of the wall of the uterus which form the menstrual cycle. These changes, like so many aspects of growth, are under the control of the endocrine system, in particular the ovary and the anterior lobe of the pituitary, and have the purpose of providing every month a fresh epithelium suitable for the reception of the fertilized ovum.

The uterine lining (endometrium) at the end of menstruation consists of a thin layer, in which are found the stumps of the uterine glands (Fig. 9.3). Under the influence of oestrogens produced by the developing ovarian follicle, the epithelium of these glands rapidly regenerates and spreads over the whole

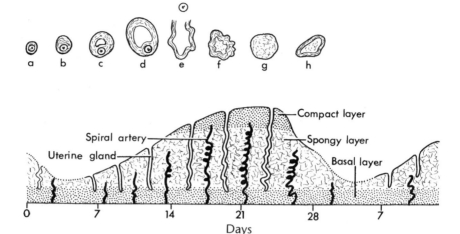

Fig. 9.3 Ovarian and menstrual cycles. The phases of the development of the ovum are shown above, while the phases of the uterine cycle corresponding to them are indicated below.

(a) Primary oocyte. Uterine mucosa being shed in menstuation.

(b) Development of follicle. Mucosa beginning to grow.

(c) Appearance of cavity in follicle. Uterine glands developing from stumps left in basal layer.

(d) Secondary oocyte surrounded by mature follicle. Glands enlarged but not yet tortuous: mucosa thickening.

(e) Follicle bursts, releasing secondary oocyte and its coverings. Compact layer of uterine mucosa developing.

(f) Follicle full of blood clot; corpus luteum forming. Uterine glands now tortuous and arteries becoming spiral.

(g) Corpus luteum of menstration. Full development of uterine mucosa.

(h) Degenerating corpus luteum. Menstration begins.

surface of the uterine cavity by the end of the first week of the cycle. From the second week onwards there is spectacular mitotic activity in the endometrium, which thickens markedly; the glands enlarge, and the blood vessels proliferate. At the same time the endometrium becomes swollen with fluid retained under the influence of oestrogens.

After ovulation, the corpus luteum secretes progesterone, and under its action the glandular cells of the endometrium enlarge, accumulate glycogen and fatty material, and begin to secrete. The glands become tortuous and dilated, and the endometrium thickens still further, until it forms three recognizable layers. The innermost layer is relatively compact, the middle layer is filled by intensely tortuous 'corkscrew' glands and by large spirally arranged arteries, so that it is called the spongy layer, and the basal layer remains much as it was at the beginning of the cycle. At the same time, the muscular wall of the uterus becomes engorged with blood and begins to exhibit rhythmic contractions.

Eventually, just before menstruation starts, changes in the balance of endocrine stimulation lead to a diminution of the extracellular fluid and the spiral arteries constrict. This deprives the superficial layers of the endometrium of their blood supply, and they are shed into the uterine cavity. The constriction of the arteries relaxes at intervals during menstruation, and thus contributes to the bleeding, which is probably mostly the result of the tearing across of veins.

This cycle has been described in some detail because it illustrates what a complicated process a growth cycle can be, and because it affords perhaps the best example of extremely rapid growth and repair occurring under normal conditions in the intact human body.

Growth cycles take place in virtually every tissue and system, with the notable exception of the central nervous system. The only difference between them and the ones described is that much less is known of the details, and that information is only now coming to hand. For instance, it was formerly thought that cells which were highly specialized had little capacity to divide and grow. A good example was the liver, in which the cells have specialized biochemical functions, and it was believed that replacement of these cells could not occur. However, it has now been shown that there is a turnover of liver cells, although the mitotic index is relatively low. Liver cells grow, divide, become old, and die, only to be replaced by new cells, so that the size and weight of the organ shows little alteration throughout adult life. The average life of a liver cell has been estimated at about 18 months.

Regeneration

After an injury greater than that imposed by normal wear and tear, the local cells are stimulated to divide until the injury is repaired as far as possible. The nature of the stimulus is unknown, although it is thought that the injured cells may produce chemicals which initiate the sequence of events concerned in healing. As cells are better at dividing in young children than in adults, it is, theoretically at least, an advantage to be a child when repairing tissue damage.

The ideal arrangement would be for a complete 'dedifferentiation' of the local tissue cells to take place, so that they reverted to their embryonic condition and could then reproduce all the various kinds of tissue which were destroyed by the injury. This is a power possessed by many lower animals, but it has been lost by higher animals somewhere in the course of evolution. It is conceivable that medicine in the future may enable us to recover it.

Animals such as *Hydra* and flat worms can grow entire new bodies from a fragment of the old one. Starfish can regenerate a limb from a body or a body from a limb. Lobsters can also regenerate a limb, although the new claw is always smaller than the original one; each time a limb is lost, the regenerating power diminishes. Fish can grow new fins, and lizards new tails.

In the early stages of regeneration of a limb or tail, phagocytic cells remove debris from the site, and large numbers of connective tissue cells and fibres appear, accompanied by blood capillaries. During this preliminary phase there is a destruction of protein and an excretion of nitrogen; this appears to be an essential part of the process whereby 'rejuvenated' and 'dedifferentiated' cells are produced.

After about a week the connective tissue cells are replaced by an accumulation of relatively undifferentiated cells, derived from connective tissue, muscle, and cartilage in the vicinity. These cells are surrounded by intercellular matrix, and multiply rapidly, forming what is called a blastema. Later still, they differentiate again into muscle, cartilage, etc., and a new limb or tail grows in much the same way as it did in the embryo. During this second phase, protein is built up and an adequate amount of dietary protein is essential.

The whole of this process appears to require the presence of a certain density of sensory innervation, and the influence of intact nerve fibres is particularly important during the phase in which the blastema forms and becomes differentiated. The nerve fibres that grow out and invade the regenerating stump are different from normal adult nerve fibres, and contain tubules which could conceivably serve to conduct to the site chemicals elaborated by the cell body. The importance of the local innervation is demonstrated by experiments on frogs. Normally, an adult frog cannot grow a new limb, although a tadpole can. But if the front leg of a frog is amputated and the sciatic nerve is simultaneously transplanted from the hind limb into the forelimb stump, a new (admittedly imperfect) limb can be regenerated. It is the sensory innervation that is vital; if the sensory ganglia are destroyed before transplanting the nerve, the limb fails to regenerate. The rate of regeneration, like the rate of growth, appears to decline with age, and shows the same variation with seasons. Vitamins, hormones, and other factors influencing growth have similar effects in relation to regeneration. Regeneration of this kind is sometimes called 'major regeneration' on the assumption that it involves true dedifferentiation of cells to a multipotent stage, so that a cell derived from one tissue can give rise to cells characteristic of another. This may be distinguished from 'minor regeneration' in which there is no evidence of such drastic preliminary dedifferentiation, and in which each tissue has to make good its own losses by the mere stimulation of mitosis.

In humans, as in other mammals, major regeneration does not occur, but minor regeneration follows the infliction of a wound or other destructive process. What is possible can best be illustrated by concrete examples, and the most obvious one with which to begin is an injury to the skin.

Repair of skin

When the skin is injured, for example by the surgeon's knife, the region of damage is immediately occupied by a blood clot. Following this there is a delay, which probably corresponds to the initial delay phase of animal regeneration, and is an essential preparation for subsequent events. In a short time, scavenging macrophages appear at the margins of the clot, having migrated out from the intact connective tissue surrounding the injury. They invade the clot and begin removing it, increasing in size as they do so because of the amount of material they ingest.

Immediately following these scavenging cells are the first new blood vessels. These are formed from the lining cells of intact blood vessels at the margin of the wound, and resemble capillaries very closely. The little sprouts grow steadily into the clot, and are at first solid; later they become canalized, join up with each other, and convey blood through the loops thus formed. Later still, smooth muscle cells appear and surround the largest of the developing vessels, which in this way are transformed into arterioles; they then acquire an outer coating of 'adventitial' cells, presumably derived from the local connective tissue. Last of all, nerve fibres invade the region and seek out the muscle cells of the new vessels, thereby providing them with vasomotor control.

A similar series of outgrowths occurs from the local lymphatic capillaries, but there appears to be no communication between the lymphatics and the blood capillaries, as was formerly supposed. The stage is now set for the production of the collagen fibres which will heal the wound and maintain its tensile strength. The exact process by which this occurs is still a matter of debate, but it is thought that the fibroblasts in the surrounding connective tissue are stimulated to divide and then to invade the clot about the same time as the blood vessels. This fibroblastic activity is perhaps the most striking feature of a healing wound. The production of collagen fibres takes time, and in animals the first of them do not appear until about 6 days after the fibroblasts invade the clot. Most of the collagen is laid down during the second week of healing, and the tensile strength of the wound increases as the collagen fibres grow and increase in number. Elastic fibres are regenerated somewhat later than the collagen fibres, but the details of this process are almost wholly unknown.

Meanwhile, the epithelial cells at the side of the wound migrate sideways on to the surface of the clot and newly formed tissue. Some cells move down into the incision, but as healing proceeds these ingrowths are discouraged and the intrusive cells are removed. Sometimes epithelial cells are driven down into the dermis at the time of infliction of the injury, and there they may form small clumps of epidermal growth which give rise to an 'implantation cyst'.

Epithelial cells are not normally motile, and what causes them to move across an injured surface has not yet been explained. It may be that a common chemical stimulus encourages both motility and the subsequent outbursts of mitosis among the epithelial cells. The mitotic index in the epithelium surrounding the wound rises to a figure about 20 times as great as that for normal skin. Initially, mitoses are found only in the normal tissue round the edges, but later the migrating cells begin to divide and mitotic figures can be seen on the surface of the injured area.

When the epithelium migrating from one side of the wound meets epithelium migrating from the other, migration ceases, and here again we do not know why, although it is commonly believed that the physical contact between adjacent epithelial cells is the stimulus. In the initial stages following the establishment of contact, the layer of epithelium covering the clot and the underlying repair processes is only one cell thick, but later it thickens until a reasonably normal cover is obtained. Structures such as hairs and sweat glands may not be completely replaced, and the new epithelium may lack the normal patterning of the skin, so that it looks shiny and glazed. If the area of a skin wound is more extensive, 'granulation tissue' develops. The base and edges of the wound swell from the accumulation of fluid and cells from the damaged blood vessels. Later, blood vessels invade the clot and debris, and the whole raw surface becomes red and granular in appearance. Each granulation has a core of delicate new blood vessels which bleed easily. The new tissue increases in thickness until the defect is filled (Fig. 9.4). Usually, this process stops when the granulations reach the level of the surrounding skin, but occasionally they proceed to bulge beyond this level, producing 'exuberant' granulations. Exactly similar events occur in granulation tissue as have already been described: invasion by capillaries is followed by invasion by fibroblasts, and eventually collagen is formed.

In the early stages of the healing of both kinds of wound the collagen can be stretched by tensile forces, but in the process of scar maturation, which may take several months, the collagen fibres increase in number and become orientated so as to resist local stretching forces. At the same time, some of the fibroblasts in the scar differentiate into myofibroblasts, which are contractile. This process of contraction is of great importance, as it pulls the edges of the wound together, and the collagen fibres give the resulting scar its strength.

The formation of a satisfactory surgical scar is influenced by the tension of the underlying muscles, which may produce stretching and broadening; elective incisions should always be made so that this tension is minimal.

Meanwhile there has been epithelial regeneration of exactly the same kind as in a simple incised wound. However, the process is naturally slower if epithelium has to cover an extensive defect, and the wound is much longer in healing completely. If some epithelial structures are left intact or only slightly

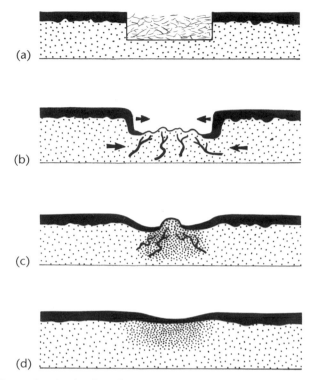

Fig. 9.4 Scheme showing healing of a granulating wound.
(a) Condition after infliction of wound, showing loss of tissue and blood and debris on the surface.
(b) Blood vessels have invaded the debris and granulations are formed. The arrows indicate invasion of the dermis by fibroblasts and also ingrowth of epidermis to cover the raw surface.
(c) Healing nearly complete. Scar tissue forming in the dermis.
(d) Complete epithelialization. Note that the epidermis is usually thinner and that its deep aspect is smoother than normal. Scar tissue in dermis.

damaged in the base of the wound, such as hair follicles or sweat glands, the epithelia of these structures will also be stimulated to divide, and little islands of epithelialization will be formed from which the surrounding granulation tissue is eventually covered. The epithelium becomes adherent to the growing granulations, and this stops their further growth, but the mechanism is again unknown.

This brief description of what happens in a simple skin wound may serve to indicate the extent of our ignorance regarding the simplest problems of growth and repair. Nevertheless, considerable advances in the understanding of local growth promoting agents will allow us to develop new concepts of processes involved in wound healing. Certainly, local hormonal messengers influence the invasion and proliferation of the repair organization and clearly if these important stimuli can be harnessed, it might lead to new methods of surgical repair to the skin and other tissues.

A good blood supply is necessary for healing to proceed normally, and it is often said that wounds of the face heal more quickly than wounds of, say, the foot because the face has such an excellent blood supply. Experimental evidence for this belief is lacking, as is evidence to support the other common statement that wounds of areas exposed frequently to injury heal more quickly than wounds of more protected areas of skin. Animal work suggests that intensities of ultrasound too low to produce a rise of temperature can stimulate tissue repair and increase the formation of blood vessels. The presence of infection in the injured tissues, or the inclusion of irritant substances in the wound area, may delay healing greatly, and if there is a general disease present, such as diabetes, the ability of the tissues to respond to the emergency may be impaired.

Although age is a factor in cell division, wounds in old age heal reasonably well provided that there is no disease of blood vessels. A good balanced diet is desirable, but minor protein deficiency has comparatively little effect, for protein seems to be diverted preferentially to the healing wound. A severe deficiency causes delay in healing. A lack of vitamin C has little noticeable effect on the regrowth of epithelium, but the formation of collagen is inter-fered with, and wounds may break down because of their poor tensile strength.

Zinc is needed for normal healing. Concentrations of zinc increase preferen-tially at the site, and zinc sulphate added to the diet of experimental animals promotes wound healing, although no histological reason for this finding can be adduced. A curious observation made in rabbits after the infliction of a small whole-thickness punched wound in the ear is that tissue regeneration in such circumstances is faster in males than in females. The effect is general rather than local, and treatment with testosterone stimulates regeneration in the female. Conversely, removal of the testes from a male rabbit is followed by a decreased rate of regeneration, provided the operation is carried out some time before the infliction of the wound.

Finally, hormones derived from the adrenal and pituitary glands can be shown to influence the healing of experimental wounds in animals, but it is questionable whether this can be of much importance in human, as only a severe disturbance produces an effect.

Repair of fractures

When a bone is broken, just as when skin is damaged, there is haemorrhage at the site of injury. This is penetrated by macrophages, and later by fibroblasts, which lay down collagen in the gap between the broken ends, so providing a

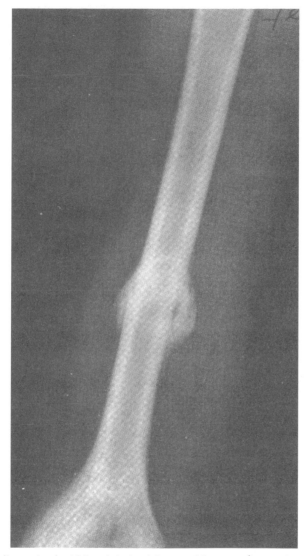

Fig. 9.5 Radiograph of middle of shaft of fractured humerus (in good position) showing the formation of provisional callus. The subsequent course of events would be roughly indicated in Fig. 9.6.

scaffolding on which calcium salts are deposited. At the same time, the bone-forming layer of the periosteum, which the injury may have displaced some little distance away from the shaft of the bone, starts to form new bone in the tissues surrounding the break (Fig. 9.5). While this is going on, other cells are producing matrix within which stem cells from the periosteum differentiate into either cartilage-forming or bone-forming cells. In some

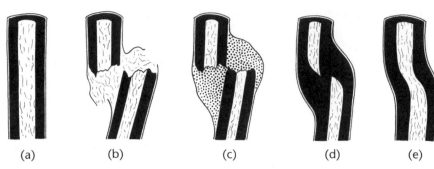

(a)　　　　　(b)　　　　　(c)　　　　　(d)　　　　　(e)

Fig. 9.6 Healing of fracture.
(a) Normal long bone.
(b) Situation immediately after break. There is a displacement and angulation of the fragments; the periosteum has been torn and displaced, and there is haemorrhage between and around the fragments.
(c) The torn ends of the periosteum have united, and the osteogenic layer is laying down bone outside the break. At the same time osteoblasts are producing bone in the region of the marrow cavity.
(d) The broken ends are united by a clumsy but efficient bridge of bone.
(e) The unnecessary new bone has been removed. In the final arrangement the architecture of the bone depends on the stresses to which the region is subject as a result of the altered mechanics of the healed bone.

instances, cartilage is formed in large amounts, but in others bone formation predominates from the beginning. In either case, the cartilage is ultimately converted into bone, which is called provisional callus.

In the initial stages, bone is laid down more or less at random in the vicinity of the break, but later, moulding takes place, and the stresses and strains around the fracture cause trabeculae to be laid down in a definite pattern. Unwanted bone is then removed by osteoclasts brought to the site by the blood vessels, and eventually a more streamlined structure is formed, which may restore the original line of the bone extremely well (Fig. 9.6). This whole process may take months or even years, but the healing of the fracture produces a structure adapted to resist the new forces which may be brought to bear on the bone if the fragments do not unite in precisely the same alignment as they had before the break.

In a child, the correction of a badly set fracture of the wrist, even one with a malalignment of as much as 60°, may be complete in 3 months, and this raises the question of the control of such healing, for it implies the existence of a 'model' of the proper shape for each part of the body; the part must be restored to correspond as nearly as possible to this model. Similarly, in attempting to straighten out a club-foot the surgeon finds that the foot is always 'trying' to return to its distorted shape, and it has been suggested that in such cases the 'model' is a distorted one. No one yet knows whether such 'models' are the expression of some process in the central nervous system, such as pattern generators, or whether they are inherent in every cell of the body.

The healing of a fracture, like that of a skin wound, requires protein and vitamin C, but in addition depends on adequate supplies of mineral salts such as calcium phosphate, normal amounts of parathormone, trace elements such as manganese and probably many other factors. Vitamin deficiencies produce characteristic differences in the healing process. Occasionally, union of the fragments does not take place, and a false joint is formed (Fig. 9.7). If healing does not take place, resulting in malunion, the application of electrical fields to the affected bone often results in renewal of the healing process and

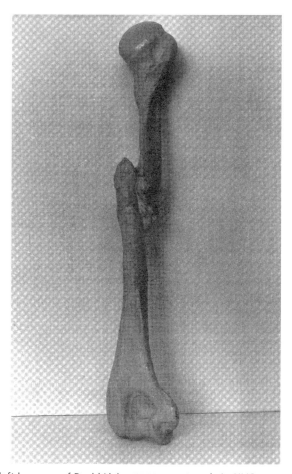

Fig. 9.7 The left humerus of David Livingstone: a cast made in 1874, some years after it was fractured by the bite of a lion. Despite the production of much callus, the fragments did not unit, and a false joint was formed. The upper portion of the shaft is greatly thinned and there is a considerable rotation deformity. (From the WMMS collections in the Wellcome Tropical Institute, by kind permission of the Trustees of the Wellcome Trust.)

reunification of the fracture; why this process works remains obscure.

After fractures of the lower limb it is usual to find a small over-growth of the bone concerned. This is of the order of 1 cm for the femur and 0.3 cm for the tibia. The disparity may continue throughout the remaining period of growth.

Repair of other tissues and organs

The nervous system

Nerve cells cannot divide to replace themselves, but, following injury to the central nervous system, attempts are made at regeneration by the supporting connective tissue cells, which behave in much the same way as fibroblasts do in the repair of injuries elsewhere. The damaged region is ultimately replaced by scar tissue, and functional deficiencies produced by cell destruction in the central nervous system are thus permanent. The presence of inhibiting factors is a major factor here.

Muscle

Human striated muscle is much less capable of regeneration than the muscle of amphibians, which has been more intensively studied. Still, a certain amount of destruction of muscle in humans can be made good. The dead tissue is removed as usual by the action of macrophages, and new fibres are derived from the satellite cells at the margins of the dead area. It is important that the connective tissue tubes which acted as sheaths for the original fibres should remain intact, so that the new fibres can grow along these tubes. The main factor which hinders regeneration of striated muscle in humans is the relative ease with which scar tissue can be manufactured. Connective tissue cells are much better at repair work than satellite cells, and scar tissue between the specialized cells obstructs their progress and closes the tubes off, before the satellite cells have had time to produce many new muscle cells.

Cardiac muscle has virtually no capacity for repair and regeneration, and any portion of the heart wall which dies following a blockage of its blood supply is repaired by fibrous tissue.

Joints and tendons

Regeneration of tendon can be reasonably satisfactory, but full functional recovery of a completely severed tendon is unusual, as the cut ends tend to unite, not only with each other, but also with the local connective tissue, so limiting movement. Articular cartilage which has been damaged may become converted into fibrous tissue. But if it is detached from the end of the bone and can find a protected region in the synovial cavity it may survive and even grow, being nourished by the synovial fluid. The knee joint, with its liability to injury and its extensive synovial cavity, is particularly prone to harbour such pieces of cartilage.

Other tissues and organs

Small blood and lymph vessels are capable of complete and rapid repair, and a damaged lymph node can reconstruct itself, although if one is completely removed it is not replaced except in young animals.

Regeneration of internal organs such as the pancreas, the salivary glands, and the endocrine glands is limited, although it is possible that given favourable conditions these organs can replace themselves better than is at present supposed. Although renal epithelium can repair itself fairly well, the kidney compensates for loss of kidney tissue by hypertrophy of the remaining tissue as well as by cellular replacement. On the other hand, the urinary bladder is remarkably efficient as regards regeneration. The lungs cannot regenerate if damaged, although lung tissue will expand to fill up the cavity left by the removal of a lobe or segment.

The internal organ which has been subjected to most investigations is the liver, for in both animals and humans it can regenerate to a quite extraordinary extent following injury or damage produced by disease. It does not seem to matter which part of the liver is removed; regeneration proceeds equally well from the remaining material, and the lobular structure of the liver is preserved in the newly formed mass. The maximal rate of liver regeneration in animals is not far short of the rate of growth in the embryo of the same species, and it has been estimated that in the first 10 days of regeneration following partial removal of the human liver as much as 100 g of liver tissue may be added each day; after the first 2 postoperative weeks there is little further change in the size of the liver remnant.

The control of liver regeneration raises many questions. For example, it is known that the body can get along quite well with only a fraction of the normal amount of liver tissue. If so, why should the liver start manufacturing new cells when there is no immediate need for them? In young, actively growing rats the restoration of the liver mass may actually exceed the original provision, often by as much as 50%.

Again, what is the stimulus which causes regeneration to take place? And how does the body know when sufficient liver tissue has been formed, so that regeneration comes to a halt? These questions are similar to those already asked regarding the repair of a skin injury, and they have as yet no definite answers, although it is possible that a chemical feedback mechanism of chalone type may be involved.

Nor is it known whether the goal of the repair process is the restoration of a critical morphological mass or the restoration of a reserve of physiological function. In the embryo, growth of organs occurs even though they have not yet begun to function; presumably this phase of growth is under genetic control, and is not mediated by physiological requirements. After birth, the situation seems to change. In some tissues and organs, such as the liver, the blood cells, and possibly the ovary, complete restoration of the original mass can occur, whereas in others, such as somatic muscle and nervous tissue, almost no attempt at specialized repair is made. To account for these findings a feedback mechanism based on functional demand has been postulated. Attempts have been made to find out whether artificial restoration of tissue mass influences repair. For example, following partial removal of the liver, the original mass of liver cells has been made up by injecting homogenates; the results have been conflicting. Transfusion of erythrocytes depresses haemopoiesis in patients with anaemia, but this may be due to factors other than the restoration of the erythrocyte mass.

Another interesting problem is presented by the difference between the repair of a local injury such as a skin wound, in which the activity is also strictly local, and the condition of compensatory hypertrophy following re-moval of one of a pair of organs, such as the kidney. In such cases the enlargement of the remaining organ requires the postulation of some generally distributed influence which affects only the 'target' organ, as generalized overgrowth of other tissues does not occur. It is difficult to escape the conclusion that this influence is the functional stress placed on the surviving member of the pair.

Regeneration of peripheral nerve

The lack of functional repair in the central nervous system must be contrasted with the results of injury to the peripheral nerves, which are composed of the processes of nerve cells. The injury in this case does not involve the nuclei of the damaged cells, and there is little difficulty in replacing the cytoplasm which has been destroyed, just as an amoeba can make up for the loss of a pseudopodium. Indeed, quite apart from any injury, the cell body is constantly synthesizing protoplasm which passes slowly down the various processes of the cell to make good the wear and tear on the protein systems they contain.

After section of a peripheral nerve, the portions of the individual nerve fibres that have been cut off from their parent nerve cells split up into small fragments, die, and are removed by macrophages which penetrate the nerve from the local connective tissue. At the same time the myelin sheaths in the nerve disintegrate into fatty globules, which are similarly removed. The result is that the nerve beyond the point of section comes to consist of a series of tubes which are cleaned out ready for the regeneration of the fibres to take place. This it does at the rate of about 1–3 mm/day with material synthesized in the cell body travelling down the fibre towards the periphery. This may sound quite fast, but it means that after a section of the sciatic nerve in the buttock it may be anything up to 3 years before the growing fibres reach the foot. Even if nothing goes wrong, the repair of a nerve injury is a slow process.

The injury to the nerve produces the usual haemorrhage between the cut ends of the nerve trunk, and this clot is penetrated and organized in the usual manner by macrophages, blood vessels, and fibroblasts. Accordingly, when the regenerating nerve fibres try to find their way across the gap they are confronted by a dense thicket of cells, collagen, and matrix which it is very difficult for them to penetrate. Those which do penetrate enter a tube to the farther stump which may or may not be the one which they formerly occupied. (As there may be several thousand fibres in the nerve, the likelihood of any one fibre reaching its former tube is pretty small). Other fibres do not succeed in getting through the obstacle, and double back on themselves, or else skirt round the scar tissue, being guided into the peripheral stump, if they reach it at all, by what appears to be a chemical stimulus.

As a result of all this activity, many fibres do succeed in getting into the peripheral stump, although very few of these are guided by the empty tubes to their original or correct destination (Fig. 9.8). Should a motor nerve fibre reach a sensory end-organ, or vice versa, it degenerates and disappears. A fibre which reaches an appropriate destination is at first much thinner than normal, but when it establishes a connection with a suitable end-organ the fibre thickens and the fibre/end-organ complex begins to function. The probability is very great that the end-organ reached will not be the same as the one originally supplied by that particular fibre, and a complicated programme of re-education in the central nervous system is therefore necessary. For example, if the patient wishes to move the little finger after section of the ulnar nerve, and if several of the fibres which originally helped him to do so have found a new destination in one of the small muscles of the thumb, it is disconcerting for him to find that his willed movement of the little finger actually causes contraction of the thumb muscle. Re-education can do something to overcome this, but good functional results can only be expected in children who have not yet established rigorous central patterns of movement.

While the regeneration process is under way, other events take place in the periphery. Many nerves that supply skin have an 'autonomous zone' which is supplied by that particular nerve and by no other. Around this central area lie the 'overlap zones', which are also supplied by one or more of the adjacent nerves (Fig. 9.9). If such a cutaneous nerve is cut, it results in an area of skin

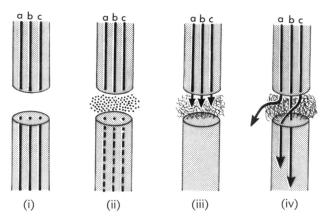

Fig. 9.8 Regeneration of nerve fibres.
(i) Situation just after section of the nerve. Three of the cut fibres in it are indicated diagrammatically.
(ii) Blood clot and debris occupy the space between the cut ends and the peripheral parts of the fibres are degenerating.
(iii) The peripheral stump has been cleared of the remains of the degenerated fibres and is ready to receive those which are beginning to regenerate. The clot has become converted into fibrous tissue.
(iv) The fate of the three fibres: (a) has failed to penetrate the connective tissue barrier and is growing into the tissues outside the peripheral stump altogether; (b) has succeeded in growing along its own peripheral tube (a rare event) and will establish its former connections once again; (c) has found its way into the peripheral stump, but has become diverted into a tube other than its own.

anaesthesia surrounded by a region in which partial sensation persists, as some of the fibres supplying this zone are still active. However, the zone of partial anaesthesia begins to shrink shortly after the injury as a consequence of the ingrowth of sprouts from the peripheral ends of the adjacent intact nerve fibres. It appears that some stimulus arising in the denervated area causes them to grow in to try to make good the deficiency.

When the fibres of the regenerating nerve arrive at the denervated zone, the invaders from the periphery tend to degenerate and be removed. One could imagine that there was some mathematical formula regarding the density of innervation desirable in a given area of skin. If this density is reduced, fibres grow in to try to make it up again; when the desirable figure is exceeded, excess fibres are removed. How this process is controlled we have no idea.

Nerve fibres invade skin grafts in a similar manner, and eventually the grafts attain a measure of sensitivity. Scar tissue is also invaded by sensory fibres, but because of the density of the tissue it is difficult for them to make their way through it. Innervation of scar tissue is therefore never completed up to 'normal' density, and the nerve fibres tend to be isolated from each other.

Nerve fibres can be extended far beyond their original length by deliberately misdirecting them. Fibres from one nerve can be induced to grow into the degenerated peripheral stump of another, and once regeneration has reached

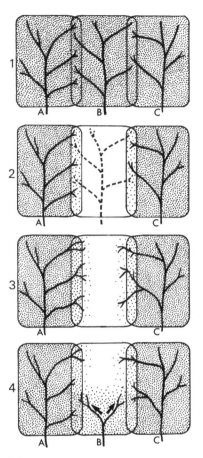

Fig. 9.9 Reinnervation of skin.
1. Patch of skin showing normal overlap of three nerve territories (other overlapping territories are omitted for the sake of clarity).
2. When the nerve B is cut, sensation is completely lost in its autonomous zone, but in the overlap zone a degree of sensation persists due to the intact overlapping nerve terminals.
3. Following degeneration of the nerve, the area of complete sensory loss shrinks, because sprouts from nerves A and C invade the autonomous zone of B. Sensation in the overlap zone also improves.
4. When the cut nerve regenerates, these sprouts regress in proportion as the normal anatomy is restored. If adequate recovery of nerve B does not occur, the sprouts persist, and the condition in diagram (3) becomes permanent. The amount of ingrowth is limited, and, unless the denervated area is very small, can never make up completely for the loss.

a certain stage this nerve can in turn be cut and introduced into the stump of the first one again (Fig. 9.10). In this way fibres will grow to very considerable lengths, and the question is at once raised: What makes the nerve fibre stop growing when it reaches a suitable end-organ? It is clear that the end-organ must in some way influence the growth of the nerve fibre and this will be by means of a local chemical neurotrophic messenger or growth promoting agent.

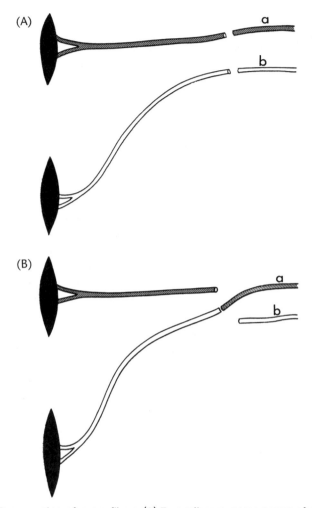

Fig. 9.10 Regeneration of nerve fibres. (A) Two adjacent motor nerves of similar size are cut: (a) supplies a muscle close to the nervous system; (b) supplies one twice as far away. (B) The central stump of (a) is sewn to the peripheral stump of (b). The fibres in (a) regenerate along the pathway provided for them by (b) and establish a functional connection with the muscle formerly supplied by (b), having grown to approximately twice their original length. If the central stump of (b) is sewn to the peripheral stump of (a) the regenerating fibres in (b) will establish a functional connection with the muscle formerly supplied by (a) and will then stop growing, though they will have travelled only half their original length.

The process of peripheral nerve regeneration is a striking illustration of growth of a cell following an injury which does not destroy the nucleus. It might be thought that this would be a much simpler affair than growth that involves cell replacement and the organization of several different tissues, but even this brief account must have shown that there are many problems which are still unsolved.

10   Disturbances of growth

Deformed, unfinished, sent before my time
Into this breathing world scarce half made up
Shakespeare

General disturbances

There are many different conditions which are associated with short stature. While some of these conditions are rarities, others are fairly common and important and demand medical attention These can include chronic disease of the kidneys or deficiencies in the capacity of the gut to absorb certain foodstuffs, a group called malabsorption diseases. Short stature is usually defined as a height below the third centile line for age on the Tanner Whitehouse chart.

Two genetic causes of disordered growth have already been mentioned: Turner's and Klinefelter's syndromes, both of which result from anomalies affecting the sex chromosomes. A patient with Turner's syndrome may suffer from a variety of local growth disturbances, some of which, such as pigmented birth marks and webbing of the neck, may be of little functional importance, whereas others, such as abnormalities of the heart or of the kidneys, may threaten life. Indeed, such figures as are available indicate that the mean lifespan of patients with Turner's syndrome is considerably reduced.

Achondroplasia

Less common than either Turner's or Klinefelter's syndromes is the condition of achondroplasia, occurring with a rate of about 1 in 10000, in which the growth in length of the long bones of the limbs is markedly impaired, although skeletal maturation is normal. The skull and trunk develop normally, and so do the muscles; the resulting distortion of normal body proportions is striking (Fig. 10.1). The basic defect in achondroplasia is inherited as a Mendelian dominant consequential to a mutation in the gene that codes for fibroblast growth factor receptor 3 (FGFR3). Achondroplastics have perfectly normal intelligence and are still often employed in the circus and on the stage.

Down syndrome

Down syndrome results from a triplication of autosome 21, so that the patient

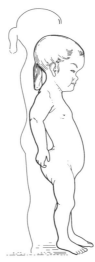

Fig. 10.1 Classical achondroplasia with features of short limb dwarfism, lumbar lordosis and a bulging skull. The outline shows a normal child for comparison.

has a set of chromosomes totalling 47 instead of 46. Its incidence at birth is about 1 in 700, although many more do not survive to term. The incidence is related closely to maternal age and pregnancy. The head is small, the eyes are slanting and slit-like and there are small ears; the tongue is large, and there are often defects in the circulatory system, particularly of the heart, and sometimes in the bones and joints of the cervical spine. Although the brain may fail to develop properly, Down children can show a wide range of intellectual skills and may have relatively advanced social skills. Most are happy and very affectionate. Other defects may include short stature or stunting of the whole body; the skeletal maturity is normal, but the teeth tend to erupt later than usual, and such children often die young. If they survive, they become adults with a reasonable life expectancy; something like half of all patients who survive infancy now live until the age of 60. Sadly, most of the survivors develop Alzheimer's disease in later late, thought to be due to the effects of genes coded to produce a protein associated with this condition on chromosome 21.

Other genetic conditions affecting growth

A much more unusual condition is cleidocranial dysostosis, which affects the bones which are ossified wholly or partly in membrane. Very little is known about its causation, although it is considered to be a dominant genetic condition. The middle portion of the clavicle, the bones of the vault of the skull, and the mandible may be either partly or wholly deficient. When the clavicle fails to develop, the shoulders can be brought together in the mid-line in front of the body. If the vault of the skull remains soft and membranous, the underlying brain may be inadequately protected. There may be disturbances in the eruption and structure of the teeth, owing to the defective ossification of the mandible.

Some genetic abnormalities affect growth less directly. In phenylketonuria, a recessive defect in which the enzyme which converts phenylalanine to tyrosine in the liver is missing, phenylalanine accumulates in the body and is converted into abnormal metabolites. Although the child may appear normal at birth, within a year or so there are signs of retarded mental development, and if the molecular defects associated with the condition are not recognized, severe mental defect develops, associated with impaired development of the brain and skull.

Again, the condition of haemophilia, which has an X-linked (female) recessive inheritance and only affects males, may cause distorted growth because of the frequency with which haemorrhages occur in relation to joints and epiphyseal plates. Severe secondary arthritis may develop in later life.

Nutritional effects

Nutritional deficiencies may give rise to a relative failure to grow in height (stunting) as well as a reduction in body mass for height (wasting). The latter is the condition dangerous to life in famines, but it responds much better in the short term to increased intake of nutrients than does the shortness of stature. Chronic abuse and neglect to a child can also cause growth failure, a condition known as psychosocial dwarfism or the Kaspar Hauser syndrome.

Role of growth hormone

As regards the hormonal causes of growth disturbance, the most obvious possibility concerns growth hormone. If too much is circulating during the period of active growth, the patient will develop into a 'pituitary giant'. Up to the age when growth would normally cease, the proportions of the body may be relatively normal, although the growth of the limbs is relatively greater than that of the trunk. Such giants are commonly of lower than usual intelligence, and many die in or before early adult life. If a pituitary giant survives beyond this time, the action of the hormone leads to continued growth in parts of the body which are still capable of growing. The condition is known as acromegaly (big periphery), and can occur in hitherto normal adults as a rare disorder if a pituitary tumour develops after growth has stopped. The bones thicken with the hands and feet becoming spade-like and limb movements appear clumsy.

The face changes its appearance, with the jaw and nose broadening. The skin and subcutaneous tissue become thick, greasy, and coarse and vision may be disturbed. The secretion of growth hormone fluctuates more than it normally does, and responds abnormally when challenged. Untreated, acromegaly is a dangerous disease with a high mortality, particularly from coronary artery disease and heart failure.

Gigantism involves internal organs as well as bones, skin, and subcutaneous tissue, and there is a general increase in the size of organs such as the heart, lungs, stomach, etc. The gonads, in contrast, are small. Initially, the muscles are well developed, but later they become weak and easily fatigued; wasting may occur. This may result from damage to the peripheral innervation or to the muscle fibres themselves. The tongue enlarges more than the mouth, and speech becomes difficult.

Treatment of acromegaly is often controversial and complete cure is often slow, if possible at all. A synthetic analogue of growth hormone called octreotide is an advance in treatment and can result in significant reductions of growth hormone levels, although gall stones can develop due to side effects on gall-bladder function.

Pituitary dwarfism and growth hormone replacement

Pituitary dwarfism, due to a deficiency in the amount of growth hormone, is thought to occur in about 1 in 5000 children. It may be difficult to distinguish from dwarfism due to other causes, such as malnutrition, congenital heart disease, rickets, etc. The skeletal proportions are usually fairly normal, and the patient simply does not grow; the body mass index is high. The facial hair commonly fails to appear, and the face may retain its childish appearance, although the skin becomes thin and often wrinkled. There is usually normal mental development, but sexual development is frequently retarded, and often the gonads do not respond at the time of puberty. If so, the epiphyseal plates of the long bones may remain open long after growth would normally have ceased, and the possibility of inducing growth in such an individual by the administration of growth hormone is a real one.

Until recently, the only way to obtain growth hormone was by its post-mortem extraction from human pituitary glands (only the human hormone is effective in human). The use of the hormone obtained in this way has had a tragic outcome as some treated cases have now developed Creutzfeld-Jacob disease (CJD), a form of dementia considered to be caused by prion proteins present in the extracted hormone preparation as a contaminant and unrecognized at the time as a risk. Pituitary extract was withdrawn in 1985 and now, all human growth hormone is produced by genetic engineering, being given the official name of 'somatropin'. This recombinant growth hormone is expensive but has

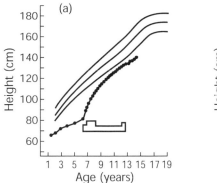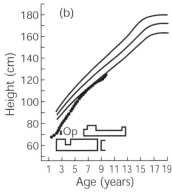

Fig. 10.2 Growth hormone deficiency. The patient's height is plotted on a cross-sectional centile chart, and in each figure the duration of treatment is shown by the linear blocks. (a) Late treatment. Catch-up growth began immediately, but the patient failed to reach the 10th centile. (b) Early treatment. The slope of the curve alters in the same way, but this time soon enough to allow the patient to catch up to the 10th centile. (From Mason, A. S. (1972) *British Medical Journal* 519–522, by kind permission of the author and the publishers).

all the effects of the natural hormone, and is used in specialist centres for the treatment of growth hormone deficient children. The results of such treatment may be striking with growth rates of between 8 and 12 cm/year being achieved (Fig. 10.2). The amount of subcutaneous fat decreases, cortical bone becomes thicker, and muscles enlarge.

The increase in height under treatment is more marked than the acceleration of bone maturation, but this is a delicate balance, and any preparation which advances bone maturation must be avoided during treatment. Patients may have to choose between delayed puberty and relatively normal height on the one hand and normal puberty and short stature on the other, for growth hormone cannot operate on closed epiphyses.

It was originally thought that treatment with growth hormone would only be of use as a replacement therapy in cases where the normal production and/or release of the hormone was depressed, and that it would have no effect on short stature due to other causes. But biosynthetic recombinant growth hormone has now been used both on short normal children with no detectable endocrine disorder and on children whose growth is impaired as a result of steroid treatment for chronic diseases, such as asthma, or as part of treatment associated with organ transplantation. Even though these results are encouraging, such studies are new and controversial and remain to be fully described. Trials in both Britain and America have increased the growth rate by 2–3 cm/year or more, with few or no side-effects; there appears to be no advance in bone age, so that the ultimate height should be improved.

However, recently, the whole rationale of treatment with growth hormone has been questioned as the major medical interest is now directed towards the achievement of a respectable final height as the therapeutic goal. It is evident that early treatment is essential. Furthermore, there is no question that replacement hormone can restore a child to normal height. Thus the big question being asked is who really needs the replacement therapy? There is little doubt of the benefits to a child who is deficient early in life as the hormone will restore some height which otherwise would not be achieved and it also has a place in the treatment of short stature in Turner's syndrome, kidney disease, and skeletal dysplasias. It is arguable whether it has any place in treating other children with short stature for questionable gains when there are risks of coronary heart disease and other problems associated with its use.

Some, but not all, growth hormone deficient children can be induced to secrete it by treatment with biosynthetic growth hormone releasing hormone, and in those that do respond the results are as good as with growth hormone itself. In such children it is likely that the defect lies in the hypothalamus, which does not produce or liberate enough growth hormone releasing hormone.

Because of the erratic and intermittent secretion of growth hormone, it is quite possible to find very low levels in normal children, depending on the time at which the sample is taken due to the cyclic nature of its release. Preferably, overnight repeated sampling during sleep is undertaken. The secretion of growth hormone is usually provoked artificially, and the response compared with that produced in normal children. Many tests have been used for this purpose: amino acids such as arginine may be injected, a protein feed such as Bovril may be given, or the patient may be made to undertake a standard exercise test. The best stimulus is the fall in blood sugar produced by an injection of insulin (insulin tolerance test), but as this is also a stressful and potentially dangerous method, it is only used in specialist centres. The response to exercise constitutes a valuable preliminary screening test. Growth hormone releasing peptides have been synthesized and are being used clinically.

The results of both tests and treatment can be assessed by measuring the amount of insulin-like growth factor (IGF)-1 (somatomedin C) in the plasma, although this is said to reflect local growth activity poorly due to multiple IGF-binding proteins giving a distorted picture of the availability of growth hormone.

As mentioned earlier, for effective treatment with growth hormone, it is essential to reach the diagnosis of growth hormone deficiency as early as possible, or otherwise the catch-up growth produced by treatment may not be adequate to allow the patient to reach a satisfactory height and treatment may well not be effective enough to be warranted (Fig. 10.2). Diagnosis should be possible by the age of 5, at which time a child with a severe degree of deficiency will have a height at least three standard deviations less than the 50th centile.

Thyroid hormone

While a deficiency or an excess of growth hormone affects the linear growth of the skeleton, a deficiency or an excess of thyroid secretion mainly affects the maturation of bone. Disorders of the thyroid gland produce either too much secretion (hyperthyroidism) or too little (hypothyroidism). The former is rare in children, but if it does occur, there is usually an acceleration of linear growth and an advance in skeletal maturation; the eruption of the teeth, on the other hand, may be slightly retarded. A hyperthyroid child who has reached the 80th centile for height may be only at the 25th centile for weight.

A severe degree of hypothyroidism that can happen when either the thyroid gland fails to form properly or the thyroid tissues develop in the wrong places, results in the patient having congenital hypothyroidism or cretinism. A cretin has severe short stature and a characteristic facial appearance; the nose is broad, the lips are thick, and the skin is thick and coarse. The skeleton to some extent retains the new-born proportions; the legs are short, and this may lead to a mistaken diagnosis of achondroplasia. The teeth erupt late, and skeletal development is held back: a normal bone age virtually excludes a diagnosis of thyroid deficiency. The retardation of skeletal growth and maturation can be completely corrected by the administration of thyroid hormone by mouth, and it is essential that this should be begun as soon as possible after birth, to prevent a permanent impairment of brain function. The intelligence of un-treated cretins is low, and there may also be defects in the development of complicated movements and of speech.

A mild degree of hypothyroidism in a child may be difficult to diagnose, and has to be considered in all unexplained cases of failure to grow. Furthermore, for normal function the thyroid depends on an adequate dietary intake of iodine, and a deficiency of iodine can cause a massive enlargement of the gland, called a goitre, and the slow development of hypothyroidism.

Thyroid deficiency in the adult leads to the condition known as myxoedema. The patient is mentally and physically sluggish, may develop a deep voice, and complains of feeling cold; these symptoms are due to the general depression of the metabolism, which also leads to an increase in weight. Disturbances of growth are evidenced by a tendency for hair to fall out and not be replaced, and a thickening of the subcutaneous tissue in the face; a characteristic loss of the hair of the eyebrows assists in the diagnosis. Many of these features are often confused with the results of ageing in older people.

Adrenal gland hormones

The cortex of the adrenal glands produces glucocorticoid hormones. An overactive cortex in childhood causes Cushing's syndrome, where the excess of glucocorticoid hormones leads to stunting of growth due to interference with the secretion of growth hormone. There is marked weight gain due to deposition of excess fat, a growth of facial hair in the female, and a typical 'moon face', which is also seen during the administration of large doses of steroids to patients as part of the treatment of other diseases such as asthma.

In contrast, the adrenal cortex may produce an excess of androgens. This condition is an autosomal recessive deficiency of an enzyme required in the synthesis of cortisol and the result is premature sexual development.

In boys, the penis, scrotum, and prostate enlarge, but the testicles may remain small and undeveloped; the secondary sexual hair appears and the voice deepens. Excess or abnormal androgen production may occur during intrauterine life, and the diagnosis of congenital adrenal enlargement (adrenogenital syndrome) may sometimes be made at birth.

In girls, the condition produces virilization; the clitoris enlarges and can be accompanied by sexual ambiguity, due to masculization of the genital organs. There is a premature development of body hair, which may follow a male pattern; the voice deepens. Menstruation and breast development do not take place.

Patients with precocious puberty of this kind are often unusually tall for their age in early childhood, and may worry about ultimate giantism. But growth stops much earlier than in normal children, and as a result the real problem is often that of short stature.

Sex hormones

Disorders of the secretion of the interstitial cells of the testicle or the ovary produce a large number of indeterminate conditions which may pose great difficulties in diagnosis. If boys are castrated before puberty, the normal accompaniments of puberty do not occur unless androgens are administered. The penis and scrotum remain small and facial hair does not appear, although there may be some pubic and axillary hair, probably as a result of adrenal activity. The voice does not 'break', and the patient becomes tall because of the delay in fusion of the epiphyses. Such patients may be either thin or fat, but usually have weak muscles: the prostate and other sexual organs remain infantile, and the thymus may persist. Typically, the lower limbs are unusually long and the trunk relatively short.

If, on the other hand. there is excess testicular secretion, skeletal maturation is accelerated, and closure of the epiphyses occurs early, resulting in small size, the legs in particular being short. Similar phenomena occur in disorders of ovarian secretion.

Insulin

Diabetes mellitus is a disease in which there is a loss of protein from the body, as it is broken down and excreted in the urine. In consequence, untreated diabetes in a child leads to a stunting of growth. This can be corrected by insulin, which has the effect of increasing protein synthesis.

Parathyroid hormone

In the adult, a deficiency of parathormone, such as may be produced by removal of one or more parathyroid glands, leads to a deficiency of calcium in the blood and an increase in the amount in the bones. On the other hand, an excess secretion of parathormone from a parathyroid tumour causes calcium to be withdrawn from the bones and renders them easily broken, for their strength depends largely on their mineral content. Excesses or deficiencies in the secretion of calcitonin in adults are not so well documented, but would be expected to be the reverse of those produced by parathormone. The effects on growth produced by alterations in parathormone and calcitonin secretion during childhood do not appear to be certainly established, but could be considerable.

Progeria

In the rare condition of progeria, the whole body is small, the sex organs remain infantile, the face resembles that of an old person, and the hair is white or absent. This is thought to be a complicated form of endocrine disorder, and has been associated with resistance to the action of insulin, but little is as yet known about it. The dental age is retarded, while skeletal and mental age are said to be normal.

Constitutional delayed growth

Despite these examples of deficiencies of hormones, organic disease is relatively unusual as a cause of general growth disturbance. Much commoner is the condition of 'constitutional delayed growth', in which delayed bone maturation is associated with delayed adolescence. In clinical practice this may be difficult to distinguish from familial short stature, in which there is no retardation of bone maturation and no delay in puberty.

There is also evidence that babies of low birth weight remain smaller throughout growth, and in such measurements as height, head circumference, and size of eyes are smaller than those whose birth weight was normal.

If referrals to a department of paediatrics on account of short stature are examined, about 60% of patients will have genetic short stature or 'constitutional delayed puberty'. The remaining 40% will be found to suffer from conditions which may include hypothyroidism, Turner's syndrome or growth hormone deficiency.

Determination of progress

Growth is a slow process, and assessing progress is therefore also slow. Because it is desirable that appropriate treatment should begin as soon as possible, velocity centile charts have a clear advantage in the early recognition of abnormal growth. Here, plotting the rate of growth can alert a paediatrician to abnormalities better than the collection of linear growth data.

A number of different anthropometric techniques have been applied to attempt to determine early information on excessive or retarded growth including very sensitive rigs for the measurement of height to accuracies of less than 1 mm and techniques to measure the segments of a limb. None of these techniques lend themselves to widespread medical and biological application and remain very much in the province of research investigation.

Local disturbances

Local disturbances of growth can be divided into congenital and acquired. Congenital deformities cover a large field of biology and medicine and so a detailed discussion is outside the scope of this book. However, by looking at a few examples, it is possible to indicate their nature.

In the first place there may be a total failure of one or more organs or parts of the body to develop, a condition known as agenesis. As an example, one or both kidneys may be absent.

More common than complete failure of local growth is a partial failure of development of an organ or tissue such as failure of vertebral arches to fuse causing spina bifida or the foramen ovale between the atria of the heart may fail to become obliterated after birth leaving an abnormal opening between the right and left sides of the heart.

Excess growth may also occur. Supernumerary nipples are not uncommon, extra digits may be produced, and a given digit may grow out of all proportion to the others (Fig. 10.3), so producing a localized 'giantism'.

Cases are also reported in which one limb may be longer than the other or one half of the body is much larger than the other half (hemihypertrophy or hemigiantism) resulting in the body appearing asymmetrical.

Tissues which normally are absorbed and removed during fetal development can also persist: for example, the baby may be born with a membrane blocking the anus. This is a condition called imperforate anus and represents the persistence of a stage in the development of the lower part of the intestinal tract. Tissues or organs may be found in abnormal situations; thus, one or more parathyroid glands, which are normally found in the neck, may descend into the chest, the thyroid gland may lie at the back of the tongue or teeth may

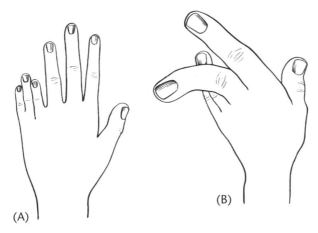

Fig. 10.3 Congenital deformities. (A) Supernumerary and (B) hypertrophied fingers. (Redrawn from Gould, G. M. and Pyle, W. L. (1896). *Anomalies and curiosities of medicine.* Julian Press, New York.)

be found in the hard palate. In the peculiar class of tumours known as teratomas, many different kinds of tissue may be found in strange situations, thus, teeth may be found in a tumour of the testicle, or stomach tissue and hair may be found in a tumour of the abdominal wall.

Finally, certain abnormalities arise through a process of fusion or of splitting. Fingers may be fused together (syndactyly), or a single horseshoe kidney may be formed; conversely, the ureter on one or both sides may be double in the whole or part of its length.

The frequency of congenital anomalies deserves particular notice. About one child in 14 that survives the period immediately following birth has a significant malformation of some kind; the incidence is much higher in children who die during this period. One-quarter of all deaths between the 28th week of pregnancy and the end of the first year of postnatal life in England and Wales are now attributable to congenital malformations. One child in 40 is estimated to have a structural defect which demands treatment. The causation of such congenital growth anomalies is still not fully understood; some are genetic, some may be due to physical conditions in the uterus, and others to events taking place during pregnancy, such as infections and chemical poisoning.

Maternal diabetes mellitus is often associated with congenital abnormalities of various kinds, and this is thought to be caused by the over-production of insulin by the fetal islets of Langerhans, as the administration of insulin can cause deformities in animals. However, rat embryos do not produce their own insulin until about the 13th day of development, and before this time they are dependent on the insulin provided by the mother. If the mother is diabetic, the low insulin levels circulating at this stage can produce abnormalities.

Viruses such as rubella or German measles can produce defects in the child if the mother contracts the disease at a time when the fetus is vulnerable, particularly in the second month of pregnancy. Vitamin deficiencies in the maternal diet, exposure of the fetus to radiation, and conditions which cause a lack of oxygenation of the blood are all possible causes. The use of drugs, both therapeutically or illegally, can affect the fetus. It was the thalidomide disaster which alerted doctors and scientists to the importance of ensuring that any drugs taken by the mother during pregnancy are fully monitored. Exposure to chemicals in the environment are also claimed to affect the fetus.

Some congenital anomalies are more common than others. For example, about 20% of the population have a communication between the two atria of the heart. If this is small, it may produce no functional disturbance whatever, and affords an excellent example of the fact that not every anatomical abnormality is associated with a physiological deterioration. Another relatively common condition (2% of the population) is a persistence of the ileal (Meckel's) diverticulum; this is usually only discovered post mortem, although it may become inflamed during life and mimic acute appendicitis. The relative clinical importance of congenital abnormalities thus varies enormously.

Some congenital anomalies are incompatible with survival such as the failure of the brain to develop (anencephaly). Other conditions cause death without urgent medical intervention. For example abnormal kidney development might require a transplant or an imperforate anus be surgically treated. Others, although not necessarily fatal, are dangerous to life or health, such as a failure of the mandible to develop properly (micrognathia) or the presence of a cleft palate. These interfere with normal nutrition because of the difficulty in sucking. Some congenital deformities of the cardiovascular system produce such an interference with oxygenation of the blood that early death may result.

In contrast, many congenital defects can be treated at leisure. Birthmarks, fusion of fingers, and the like come into this category. Indeed, a large proportion of vascular birthmarks regress spontaneously and disappear as the child gets older.

Finally, some defects which are untreatable are important and others are not. For example, agenesis of one kidney can become a vital factor if the other becomes diseased, but a condition such as the existence of bilateral brachiocephalic arteries is seldom likely to worry either the patient or his medical adviser.

One system commonly involved in congenital defects is the locomotor system, but many of the conditions which affect it are trivial; even absence of such a large muscle as the pectoralis major may produce no disability apart from the cosmetic problem. The system least affected is the respiratory system.

Some abnormalities occur at different rates in males or females. For example, congenital dislocation of the hip is seven times as common in females, adolescent idiopathic scoliosis is more common in females and a congenital enlargement of the pyloric sphincter (pyloric stenosis) is about four times commoner in males.

Many congenital defects are obvious at the time of birth and others become detectable within a few days or weeks. Hence, as we have seen, some defects can affect the survival of the new-born baby, all infants should be examined for the presence of gross congenital abnormalities by a paediatrician.

Other defects may not become apparent for a few months or even years. This is particularly true for urinary tract anomalies, which make their presence known through repeated infection of obstructed urine. In the alimentary system, developmental errors affecting the gut can present as vomiting. A deficiency in the normal development of the intrinsic innervation of the colon can result in severe constipation and an enormous dilatation of the gut (Hirchsprung's disease). Defects can also affect the bony development of the vertebral column resulting in the spinal cord being progressively damaged by the differential growth of the vertebral column and the cord itself. Consequently, the nerve roots and the cord are subject to stretching so that in later childhood or adolescence paralysis and loss of bladder control may ensue. Within this group are the congenital defects associated with some forms of scoliosis, or curvature of the spine, which can interfere with growth of the trunk and may lead to short stature in adulthood.

Hyperplasia, hypoplasia, and hypertrophy

Before proceeding to consider acquired local disturbances in growth, it is necessary to discuss some definitions. The first of these is the term hyperplasia, which is applied to a local increase in the number of cells in an organ or tissue, such as occurs in the gonads at puberty. This process is reversible; we have already seen that the hyperplasia of the blood-forming cells in the bone marrow following severe blood loss regresses again once the blood loss has been made up.

The number of cells in a unit volume of tissue can theoretically be increased in three ways. Prolongation of the life span of the individual cells, acceleration of differentiation, and an increase in the rate of cell division will all have this effect; the last is the usual way in which hyperplasia is produced.

The distinction between hyperplasia and the normal growth of cells in an adult tissue (Chapter 9) may be appreciated by considering once again the situation in the skin. The thickness of the epidermis remains more or less constant because there is an equilibrium between the rate of division of the stem cells and the rate of removal of the superficial cells. Now suppose there is an increased shedding of dead cells from the surface because of some disease process or mechanical attrition. This, by a complex chemical mechanism, of which we know very little, influences the division rate in the germinative layer so that a new equilibrium is reached. More cells are now to be found in the germinative layer than would be there in normal circumstances, and this is what is meant by hyperplasia. The converse of hyperplasia, in which fewer than the normal numbers of cells are present, is called hypoplasia.

The next term which requires definition is hypertrophy. This means an enlargement of cells without an increase in their number. Increase in the size of its component cells naturally results in an increase in the size of an organ or tissue, which is then said to be hypertrophied. Hypertrophy may result from an increased functional demand. Thus, if there is a gradually increasing obstruction to the outlet of a hollow organ, the muscle which expels the contents of the organ will hypertrophy. A narrowed valve in the heart will result in a thickening of the cardiac muscle fibres and an increase in the thickness of the wall of the chamber of the heart primarily concerned. Similarly, the wall of the bladder thickens when the urethral outlet is progressively blocked by an enlarged prostate gland. Somatic muscle can be made to hypertrophy by exercising it: the smaller fibres in the muscle are brought up to the normal average size, but those which are already large do not appear to enlarge further.

When a blood vessel is blocked, the small collateral branches which unite with similar branches of the neighbouring blood vessels enlarge to carry the blood past the obstruction (Fig. 10.4). This enlargement is progressive, and takes place over several days; the stimulus which causes it is thought to be the increase of pressure inside the small vessels, and in this case the hypertrophy of the wall is accompanied by a hyperplasia of the cells composing it. Other examples of hypertrophy and hyperplasia are seen in the uterus and the breasts during pregnancy, when they are attributable to the effects of various hormones.

Finally, a condition called compensatory hypertrophy develops when one of a pair of organs such as the kidney or the ovary is removed. The remaining kidney or ovary enlarges. The ovary may enlarge possibly even to the size of the combined mass of the ovaries before operation, and the kidney perhaps to 80% of the original combined mass. If the functional units of an organ undergoing compensatory hypertrophy are single cells, the enlargement of the whole organ may be due to hyperplasia of the active cell population, as in the adrenal cortex. If the organ contains more complicated functional units, such as the nephrons of the kidney, these cannot apparently be multiplied beyond the original normal adult complement, and a certain amount of cellular hyperplasia is supplemented by cellular enlargement, both processes resulting in a more or (usually) less complete restoration of the number of functional units and some increase in their size. In this way much of the functional

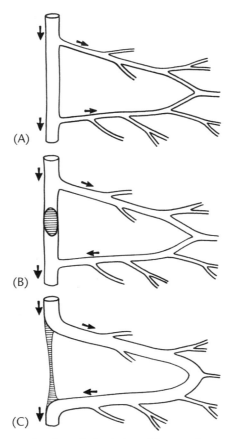

Fig. 10.4 Development of collateral circulation. (a) Normal anatomy. Little blood flows along the anastomotic connection between the two collateral branches of the artery. (b) Clot forms in the main artery between the two branches. Pressure beyond the site of blockage falls, and blood now passes through the anastomosis and back to the main trunk. (c) Revised anatomy. The main artery is permanently obliterated by fibrous tissue and shrinks to a fibrous cord. The increased pressure has caused the anastomotic channel to dilate; evantually its walls thicken by hypertrophy and hyperplasia and it becomes a vessel indistinguishable from the original main artery. The blood is now supplied to all parts of the territory formerly supplied by the main artery just as efficiently as before.

deficiency is made good, so much so that removal of 80% of the total kidney substance is not necessarily fatal. In the ovary most of the compensatory hypertrophy is the result of follicular growth and maturation, and in the testis, which does not enlarge to anything like such an extent after a unilateral removal, the increase in size is mostly due to the growth of the interstitial tissue.

In many cases the response of hypertrophy can be shown to depend on functional demand. Thus, although a congenital absence of one kidney may be accompanied by hypertrophy of the other after birth, such hypertrophy is not evident in cases of stillbirth where the kidney has never worked. Again, hypertrophy of the thyroid gland following partial removal can be prevented by the administration of thyroid extract.

Atrophy

The converse of hypertrophy is atrophy. This term is used to imply either a loss of cells or a diminution in their number, or both, and is also applicable to the consequent shrinkage of the organ or tissue in which this happens.

Atrophy may follow disuse; if a limb is immobilized in plaster of Paris and the muscles are not kept exercised by physiotherapy, they will be found to have shrunk when the plaster is removed. Malnutrition produces atrophy, as can be seen in famine victims. Lack of sufficient blood supply, as in the heart wall when the coronary vessels are becoming narrowed, can cause atrophy. Denervation of muscles results in their atrophy, for reasons which are not completely understood; it is probably due to something more complicated than simple disuse, and trophic factors may be concerned. Finally, endocrine disorders may produce local atrophies. For example, in Simmonds' disease, in which the anterior lobe of the pituitary gland is destroyed, there is a reduction in the size of the heart, with atrophy of the gonads, the adrenal cortex, and the breasts.

These facts raise once again the question of the control of growth in a normal tissue or organ. In any biological material the balance between anabolism and catabolism is the fundamental factor which determines the mass of the material at any given time, and it has already been postulated that the feedback mechanism which controls this balance is a chemical product of the active cells. But clearly the response of a tissue to increased or decreased functional demand, its reaction to denervation, and the results of endocrine disturbances, indicate that there may be other chemical mechanisms of which we know virtually nothing. Probably the range within which the balance operates is determined genetically, and within this range the chemical mechanisms constitute the 'fine adjustment'.

Another term which requires discussion is metaplasia. This means a replacement of one tissue by another; the new type is thought to come from cells which have never completely differentiated, and so have retained many of their original wide potentialities. A common type of metaplasia occurs when the ciliated respiratory epithelium in the air sinuses or the bronchi is replaced by squamous epithelium as a result of prolonged surface irritation. Another common example is the appearance of cartilage in tendons subjected to localized friction. Metaplasia is a sign which may be a precursor of cancerous changes in cells.

Malignancy and cancer

An estimated one in three people will probably develop some form of cancer during their lifetime. Cancer is an emotive word, but with recent advances in our understanding of the nature of malignancy and the behaviour of growing cells, treatment methods have improved considerably during the last decade.

Malignant growth differs from normal cell division and also from hyperplasia in that it is progressive and continues irrespective of external stimuli. This process is called neoplasia and occurs when the process of cell division within a tissue or organ becomes uncontrolled, with the result that there is a rapid increase in size of the affected tissue. This leads to the formation of a tumour or neoplasm.

If normal cells undergo an irreversible and abnormal change which affects the way they grow and divide, they can become neoplastic, transmitting their new abnormal genetic make-up with its abnormal growth-controlling mechanism to their descendants. Nevertheless, some of the characteristics of the normal tissue cells may persist in some of the members of the family. In any tumour there are many stem cells and mitotic figures are common, but some of the daughter cells become differentiated to a greater or lesser extent, and may carry out functions typical of their heritage. For example, many of the cells of a tumour derived from the thyroid gland may continue to secrete thyroid hormones.

The proportion of stem cells and relatively differentiated cells varies according to the particular tumour and the rate at which it is growing; fast-growing tumours have naturally many stem cells, but slow-growing ones may resemble normal tissue quite closely on superficial microscopical examination. One of the reasons for the excessive growth of tumours may be that the cells in the tumour do not mature and differentiate as quickly as normal and therefore remain capable of dividing for a greater proportion of their lifespan. Tumour cells do not divide any more rapidly than normal tissue cells, and their mitotic cycle may even be slower. Different tumours have very different proportions of active proliferating cells. In some the proportion may be as low as 5%, and in others as much as 100%.

Some tumours are classified as benign; that is, they do not invade the surrounding tissues, and produce their effects merely by their size and the consequent pressure on adjacent structures, or by the functional results of the activity of their differentiated cells. Other tumours become malignant, and their cells proceed to infiltrate and destroy surrounding tissues. These tumours are also capable of forming daughter tumours (metastases) in distant sites by cells becoming detached from the primary tumour and being carried away by blood vessels or lymphatics to settle elsewhere in the body. This is an unpleasant feature of malignant tumours as nests of cells are capable of further growth in new, and often apparently unsuitable, surroundings which can then hasten the death of the affected individual.

A 'two-hit' theory of malignancy has been proposed. Over-production of growth factors at the site of the future tumour is followed by the first 'hit' or mutation, which transforms one of the resulting hyperplastic cells into the progenitor of a neoplastic line of cells. This leads to the production of a primary tumour in which the cells are still dependent on the local supply of growth factors. Any cells breaking away and being carried to a distant site at this stage would die. A second 'hit' is therefore needed to allow the neoplastic cells to become independent of their growth factors, so that they could survive and multiply to form metastases.

Sometimes the cells in malignant tumours present with a totally undifferentiated structural morphology, collectively described as anaplasia. Associated with this, the orientation of the structures within the cells is often disturbed and there is a considerable range in the shape and size of the nuclei. Mitoses occur in large numbers, and are often abnormal in appearance with the chromosome number often being irregularly altered (aneuploidy). The organization of the cells into a tissue is also abnormal, with variations in structure in different parts of the same tumour. Sometimes the growth of the tumour outstrips its blood supply, and many of the cells within the tumour can then be seen to be dead or dying. In other cases there is no apparent breakdown of blood supply, and it is suggested that in such circumstances the death of cells occurs because the mass of the tumour is, like the mass of ordinary tissue, controlled by a self-regulating mechanism as yet not fully understood. Again, intrinsic errors in the abnormal cells may lead to a high wastage, and tumours which grow fast tend to have a high loss of cells.

The causes of local disturbances of growth are numerous and varied. Local growth is stimulated by injury, and occasionally the process may be rather too enthusiastic, so that more scar tissue is formed than is needed to repair the defect. If the scar tissue extends beyond the boundaries of the original wound into the normal tissues, it is called keloid. The formation of keloid is commoner during pregnancy but the reason for this is obscure. The overgrown scars which sometimes follow acne are considered by some to be a type of keloid. Very little indeed is known about the genesis of keloids, and they may appear spontaneously in uninjured skin. They occur most often on the upper part of the trunk, and never on the palm or sole.

The skin may produce an overgrowth of tissue if it is irritated, especially if the irritation is intermittent; for example, local pressure may produce a corn confined to the site of pressure. This is in one sense a kind of tumour, but there is no uncontrolled growth of the germinative layer, and the corn will regress and disappear if the irritation is removed. On the other hand if certain types of irritation are continued for too long, an uncontrollable neoplasia may be engendered, and eventually spreads beyond the site of the stimulus (local malignancy) or to distant parts of the body (general malignancy). Removal of the original irritative cause then has no effect on the further growth of the tumour.

Chemical irritants and cancers

In the eighteenth century, it was first recognized that irritation could produce cancer in workers. Cancer of the skin was observed to be common in people who worked with tar which acted as an irritant. In 1928 Kennaway discovered that 1,2,5,6-dibenzanthracene, isolated from tar, possessed the ability to induce cancer when painted on the skin. Several such carcinogens have since been identified and these act by changing the genetics of the cells, rendering them malignant. Such a situation arises with cigarette smoking which is known to be associated with cancer of the lung. The mechanism of action appears to involve reactive oxygen species, molecules present in the smoke, which attack the repair mechanisms of the cells in the respiratory tract. Individuals susceptible to cancer lack one of the genes carried on chromosome 3 called Ogg1 which acts to repair damage to cells caused by the reactive oxygen species; as a result, a build-up of faulty DNA is thought to lead to the cells becoming malignant. The same mechanism might explain why passive inhalation of cigarette smoke containing the same reactive oxygen species by non-smokers can also lead to cancer if they also lack this gene, opening them to susceptibility to develop the cancer.

Other examples of cancer which may involve this mechanism are known. Cancer of the stomach can develop after a long-standing stomach ulcer or may be induced by active chemicals in the diet. Red meat is thought to contain carcinogens. There is also concern about an apparent rise in the number of cases of bowel cancer in younger age groups; there are fears that diet may play a part in this change. Cancer of the tongue was associated with smoking a clay pipe, and cancer of the skin is common if the skin is exposed to excessive ultraviolet light in sunlight. This latter problem is increasing in northern Europeans who are unwisely sunbathing in the strong sun of southern Europe. There is also concern that it may also be linked to the depletion of the ozone layer in the atmosphere. It does not seem to matter what the irritant is; provided it is adequate to produce a neoplastic change by interfering with the DNA in cells making them potentially malignant, the subsequent course of events is similar in all cases, though the actual tumours naturally have different characteristics, because they develop from different types of cells.

Viruses, genes, and other factors

Some viruses are known to cause neoplasms and malignant conditions. A class of viruses called retroviruses have provided researchers with the first clues that have identified genes within cells which might become important in causing tumours. These are called oncogenes. The DNA of the virus can become integrated into the DNA in the host cell, causing a mutation and thus rendering it potentially malignant and capable of causing a cancer. However, the reverse process may take place with the cancer causing genes and DNA within a cell being reintroduced into the viral DNA, making the virus able cause malignant changes if it affects further cells. It is important to appreciate that these changes do not necessarily cause a neoplasm but in fact change the genetics of a cell rendering it potentially malignant. It is known that some malignant tumours of animals are caused by viruses, but it is still unclear how much this applies in causing malignant neoplasms in humans. Infection by viruses can also cause benign tumours to form such as the ordinary cutaneous wart.

The oncogene is an important genetic factor in causing abnormal cell growth which leads to cancer occurring. Cell function is upset by the oncogene causing cells to suffer from an unregulated stimulus for division due to disturbance of the normal growth control messages and possibly their excess production by the cell; one of the first oncogenes discovered which functions in this way is called ras. Cells may also be affected by oncogenes causing a loss of important functional mechanisms which in their absence result in uncontrolled cell division.

It has been the continuing unravelling of the human genome which has led to the identification of genes which seem to be present in a wide range of cancers. An example is the p53 gene found on chromosome 17 which acts by controlling cell repair and cell division. It is a mutation of this p53 gene which has been found in cancer of the bowel, lung, and breast. How the gene works in causing malignant change is still not clear, although recent work has shown it may control the growth of blood vessels, which is an important component in tumour growth as many neoplasias rely on a rich blood supply to develop.

Some malignancies have been shown to be inherited, with affected families being found to carry a cancer-causing gene. Examples of this mechanism include the recently identified genes *BRCA1* and *BRCA2*, which have been found to be associated with cancer of the breast. The genetic mechanism of how this operates is still unclear for it often takes many years for the cancer to develop. Some inherited tumours are highly malignant, such as retinoblastoma, a genetically determined tumour of the retina, which develops in early childhood. It also appears that the *Ogg1* gene which is responsible for internal repair of cellular damage is important in cancers such as lung cancer.

In contrast, other DNA sequences act as repressors of malignancy, and have been christened anti-oncogenes. Work is in progress to try to elucidate the part these genes may play in aborting the development of cancer in humans.

Other factors

Normal tissue cells also contain 'proto-oncogenes' which can be converted to oncogenes by factors within the environment called carcinogens. These can include pollutants such as pesticides, industrial chemicals and radiation. Most carcinogens are thought to operate by interfering with the cell genes in this way.

It is also recognized that there is a group of proteins known as cytokines which occur naturally in the body and have effects on both normal and tumour growth. The alpha-interferons are members of this group, and have been shown to have a direct inhibitory effect on human tumour cells. Research in this field is continually discovering agents which can affect tumour growth.

Hormones are known to influence established neoplasms of particular organs such as cancer of the prostate, which is susceptible to treatment by oestrogens. Some cancers of the breast rely on oestrogen for their development and these can be made to regress temporarily by removal of the ovaries or by using anti-oestrogen drugs such as tamoxifen. It is probable that hormonal factors may be concerned in the production of other tumours as many endocrine-related tumours contain somatostatin receptors and it has been suggested that somatostatin may inhibit tumour growth.

Radiation can also induce malignant tumours. The classic example occurred in a factory in which radioactive material was used to paint luminous figures on watch dials. The workers used to moisten their paint brushes with their lips, and in this way took in an amount of radioactive material sufficient to produce malignant tumours of their bones.

Research on cells exposed to radiation resulted in the discovery of intracellular proteins which are capable of repairing damage to their DNA. These are controlled by genes such as the *Ogg1* gene found on chromosome 3. Up to a point these proteins enable the cells to resist injury of several kinds as well as that due to radiation by taking care of general housekeeping and mopping up the damage caused by free radicals and reactive oxygen species. Clearly, they must play an important part in the defences of the body against cancer and other diseases.

Finally, the role of the mind may be important in the growth of cancers. It is well known that stress and attitude of mind can affect cancers; for example, breast cancer has been reported to be better controlled by women prepared to adapt and fight the disease while those who did not tended to have a poor outcome. Such outcomes may be mediated by the nervous system and its effects on the immune system, although the processes underlying any recoveries from cancer if they exist, remain obscure.

11   Old age

There are so few who can grow old with a good grace
Steele

Senescence

Today, the increased standards of living and associated improvements and advances in medical care are resulting in more people living longer so that the proportion of the population in the older age groups is increasing, sometimes rapidly. Age-related changes occur in the body and more and more health affecting problems can arise. Because of this, it is helpful to divide the older age groups into three groups in a widely used classification which regards those aged 60–74 as 'young old', those aged 75 and over as 'old old', and those aged 90 or over as 'oldest old'.

The reasons for the increased proportion of older people are twofold. First, there is a general reduction in fertility in the developed countries. Secondly, a decline in infant mortality as a consequence of the high standard of living is allowing more people to live through to old age. Undoubtedly, a similar change in pattern of the population will occur in other poorer countries as their socio-economic status develops in the future.

During the period 1900–80 the percentage of people over 65 in the United States rose from 4 to 11.3%, and the life expectancy of a baby born there rose from 47.3 to 73.6 years. It is now 74.6 years (78.7 for white women, 73.6 for black women, 71.7 for white men, and 65.7 for black men).

In Britain, as we approach the millennium, over 10 million people are now over the age of 65 compared with only about 2 million in 1900: the number aged over 85 has increased by 40% in the last 25 years.

However, the expectation of life of elderly and old people is not increasing as fast as that of young people. Though medical research has been able to prevent early death and to prolong the life expectancy of those in middle age, it has not solved the many problems associated with ageing.

This is due to the great difficulty still faced by science in defining ageing in biological terms and recognizing the processes associated with normal ageing as opposed to the onset of age-related disease. Most of what we all see and experience as ageing is in fact due to the accumulation of minor 'disease' processes, as true ageing still remains a universal, progressive, intrinsic, irreversible, and deleterious process, a rather depressing thought for us all!

As we get older, random biological, chemical, and cellular changes occur throughout the body and sooner or later, one of these changes causes something harmful to happen to the body. The older the person is and the longer they live, the more likely they are to be subject to a detrimental effect. Research has revealed that approximately 80% of people over 65 are afflicted with one or more chronic illnesses with the consequence that senescence and old age are more likely to be accompanied by these progressive chronic disease processes, often taking the form of a sequence of knock-on effects which eventually prove fatal.

Thus medicine cannot distinguish confidently between these inherent random changes occurring with the passage of time and those due primarily to disease. It is quite possible that there is a genetically determined 'curriculum vitae' which operates quite independently of wear and tear and of disease. It is therefore necessary to distinguish between increased life-span and increased span of activity. Figures from Canada indicate that 70% of the gain in life expectancy in men between the years 1951 and 1978, and 80% of the corresponding gain in women, consists of increased years of disability.

Just as the best way of becoming tall is to have tall parents, so the best way of becoming old is to have long-lived parents, although the correlation between longevity of parents and longevity of children is not as good as that for height. It is also very advantageous to be female, for 'old old' and 'oldest old' women considerably outnumber 'old old' and 'oldest old' men; there are probably six times as many female centenarians in Britain as there are male ones. The reason for this discrepancy is not understood, although there are many suggestions. It may be, for example, that the Y chromosome is responsible for shortening life; if so, individuals with two Y chromosomes might afford useful information, but too little is yet known of their life-span compared with normal males. It has been claimed that patients with the Klinefelter syndrome may show a female capacity for survival because they have two X chromosomes; this genetic pattern has been said to enhance synthesis of immunoglobulins and to protect against infections.

There is little prospect that in the near future centenarians will cease to be exceptional people, although it is likely that more and more of the population will survive into the octogenarian range. The maximum life-span authenticated by appropriate documentation is that of Jeanne Louise Calment in France who died at the age of 122 years, 5 months and 14 days in 1997. Records suggest only four other cases have been verified when people lived beyond 115 years. Claims of much greater ages have been made with the best known being those of Bir Narayan Chaudhary in Nepal at 141 years and a former Brazilian slave Maria do Carmo Geroniomo at 126. However, such 'really' old and long lived people have vulnerable claims to true authenticity because of poor or absent documentation and clear proof of identity.

Because of the numbers of old people, a knowledge of the structural and functional changes which occur in old age is becoming progressively more important. These changes, which are collectively known as 'senescence', do not occur to any extent in populations of wild animals, because most individuals die of disease or are killed and eaten by predators before the processes have time to develop very far. Even in the laboratory it takes an immense amount of effort to produce a senile rat. Human beings therefore have to serve as the experimental animal, and even in countries with a reasonable standard of living it is only in the latter part of this century that the average life-span has increased sufficiently for senescence to become a feature. The study of senescence is thus among the youngest disciplines of medical science.

Senescence is a stage on the pathway to death, a stage which, because of the cumulative nature of the random changes that have occurred on the way to it, increases the likelihood of death occurring. Many of these changes are due to the random biological, chemical, and cellular defects in the processes of growth and of replacement of damaged cells. Their major manifestations occur for the most part after the end of the child-bearing period, and it is therefore probable that resistance to them has not yet evolved very far. However, just as in youth the systems of the body have different growth curves, so they have different curves of deterioration. It may even be said that senescence begins to make itself felt as soon as maturity is reached, for by then the first signs of functional inadequacy are apparent in the nervous system. Natural selection could conceivably operate on these early alterations, which may render some individuals marginally less fit than their competitors.

As yet no comprehensive longitudinal studies of ageing have been published, although one is in progress in Baltimore. The difficulties of such investigations are even more formidable than those in similar studies of growth and maturation; cross-sectional data are open to the usual objections.

Ageing of cells and tissues

Changes in cells

The obvious place to look for signs of age in cells is the nervous system, as nerve cells are as old as the body to which they belong. In old age some nerve cells have irregular nuclei which stain more darkly than normal, and may contain rods and filaments not found in young cells. Shrinkage occurs in the Purkinje cells of the cerebellum and the pyramidal cells of the motor cortex, and it is likely that there is shrinkage of other cells also, although this is difficult to establish with certainty. In senile cells the Nissl substance may be depleted, and increasing amounts of a yellow-brown pigment known as lipofuscin are deposited in the cytoplasm, pushing the nucleus to one side. These 'lipofuscin bodies' may be the end-stage of cellular lysosomes which cannot get rid of their contents by voiding them from the cell, but others believe that they are derived from the degeneration of mitochondria. Similar pigment is found in old age in somatic muscle cells, the cortex of the adrenal glands, the interstitial cells of the testicle, and the lining of the male reproductive system.

The dendrites in the brain may become more complex, and short new ones may be formed; structures known as argyrophil plaques and neurofibrillary tangles may appear. All these changes are difficult to evaluate because so far there has been little effort to quantify the results, to exclude disease, and to avoid artefacts due to post-mortem changes or differences in experimental technique.

It was once calculated that the brain loses something like 10 000 nerve cells every day, and that by the age of 65 or so about 20% of the total number of nerve cells present at birth have died.

However, the evidence for a steady loss of cells is unsatisfactory, and it is now known that some at least of the nuclei of the brainstem retain their complement of cells into advanced old age. In contrast, the substantia nigra loses cells fairly rapidly. The numbers of Purkinje cells and cells in the temporal cortex remain fairly steady until the age of 60–65 years, after which they begin to decrease. In spite of these reservations, increasing age brings a diffuse atrophy of the brain, particularly in such regions as the frontal lobes. The fissures become wider and deeper, the weight of the brain declines by up to 10%, and the proportion of neuroglial tissue increases. The loss of brain weight appears to begin about a decade earlier in women than in men. In the spinal cord and posterior root ganglia pigmentation and atrophy are progressive, so that after the age of 80 few cells in the ganglia are unaffected. There is a concomitant loss of fibres in the dorsal roots, and the motor neurons of the lumbosacral cord are also reduced in number. There is probably a large reserve of neurons in the brain and spinal cord, so that a substantial loss is needed before symptoms and signs are produced.

The other tissue in which the cells have a very long life is somatic muscle, but unequivocal evidence of senile, as opposed to pathological, changes in human somatic muscle is hard to find; there are said to be alterations in the arrangement and integrity of the myofibrils, deposition of lipofuscin granules, and a relative increase in the collagen and elastin content of the muscles. Recent work with isolated mitochondria from somatic muscle has shown an impairment of respiratory function which correlates with ultrastructural evidence of mitochondrial degeneration with age. Atrophy and loss of muscle fibres leads to a decrease in the total weight of somatic muscle in the body by about 30% between the ages of 30 and 90, and there is a corresponding loss of muscle power. The average size of the surviving fibres may increase in what is possibly an effort at compensation. The relative, and perhaps the absolute, increase of connective tissue in senile muscles may be one reason why they tend to become stiff.

Many factors may combine to cause the loss of muscle tissue. Motor nerve cells die and their motor units atrophy; there may be a failure of the trophic mechanisms of the nerves supplying the muscle; the blood supply to muscle decreases, and the production of testosterone, which stimulates the increase of muscle at the time of puberty, diminishes. The generalized atrophy of somatic muscle contributes to the typical 'wasted' appearance of the very old, but this may be masked by the deposition of fat in middle age, and some old people still have a hearty appetite, with the result that their body weight may actually increase instead of decreasing. The composition of such a person's body is necessarily very different from that of a young adult.

In other tissues the cellular content also diminishes, because growth processes come to be inadequate to effect normal running repairs. Just as there is a limit to the age of an individual cell, so there appears to be a limit to the number of times the descendants of that cell can divide to form new offspring. For example, Hayflick showed that human fibroblasts have a finite performance in tissue culture; a sheet of them grown on nutritive medium will 'double' itself from 40 to 60 times, and then the cells in it will die. Cells removed from the culture after 30 such doublings and put into cold storage will, if revived, 'remember' the stage they had reached, irrespective of the time interval, and will go on to divide about 20 more times before dying. Towards the end of the lifetime of such a culture, aberrations in the chromosomes begin to show up, and there is a decline in the capacity for cell division.

On the other hand, skin from old mice transplanted into young mice of the same inbred strain can survive beyond the normal expectation of life of the donor, and there is evidence that a genetic factor is involved.

Human and animal cells have been made to grow in culture for many years. The HeLa strain of cells was derived from the uterine cervix of a patient in the USA in 1952 and is still growing, having become widely distributed throughout the world in experimental laboratories. In fact, this particular line of cells may well have become almost a problem as it seems to appear in many culture cell lines!

Cells will only acquire this long life after they have undergone changes which transform them into abnormal cells. For example, the HeLa strain came to have several hundred chromosomes per cell, and many of the so-called 'immortal' lines of animal cells will grow as malignant tumours if injected into a suitable host of the same species. Neoplastic cells are easy to grow in tissue culture, and can be maintained pretty well indefinitely.

The number of 'doublings' in tissue culture is referred to as the 'Hayflick number', and varies greatly in different species. For example, chicken fibroblasts are very stable throughout the lifetime of the culture, but mouse fibroblasts invariably become 'permanent' lines of 'immortal cells'. Humans are intermediate in this respect.

The evidence is at least suggestive that the same sort of thing happens in tissue culture happens to cells growing in their natural surroundings in the intact body, and the Hayflick number can be related, at least roughly, to the life-span of the species. Neoplastic growth is commoner in old people than in the young. At the age of 25 a man has a 1 : 700 chance of developing cancer in the following 5 years; when he is 65 the chance is 1 : 14. Yet if cancer does occur in old age, the growth capacity of the cancer cells is often less than in a younger person, and consequently such neoplasms tend to be slower growing and less invasive.

At the age of 50 the prevalence of cancer in American men is at present about half that in women, largely because of cancer of female breast. But by the age of 70 the figures for men overtake those for women, and from then on the male prevalence is greater. Cancer accounts for about 30% of deaths in people aged 69, but only about 10% of those aged 89.

The gradual loss of cells from every tissue and organ of the body inevitably produces alterations in bodily functions and chemistry among which is naturally a lowering of the basal metabolic rate. In addition, the diminished ability of cells to undertake divisions is reflected in a lessening of the ability to repair damaged tissues, or to hypertrophy in response to stress; compensatory hypertrophy in response to the removal of one kidney, for example, is relatively poor in old people.

Degeneration

Degeneration is a difficult word to define: it implies a breaking down of an organized structure to one less organized in form or in function. The problem can arise in a variety of ways in different tissues, and this makes it hard to say whether the changes are the result of old age or of disease.

Dying differentiated cells may be replaced by fat cells (fatty degeneration), or by spaces filled with fluid (cystic degeneration). In the intima of the major arteries there occurs an extremely important and common form of degeneration called atherosclerosis, in which small plaques of fibrous and fatty material protrude into the lumen of the vessel, so encouraging the formation of a clot. The term degeneration is also applied to alterations in tissue matrix which cause a simplification and deterioration of a complicated structure, such as bone or intervertebral discs.

Changes in tissue matrix

The matrix of a tissue determines such important properties as its rigidity, elasticity, and lubrication, and in old age all these properties are disturbed to a greater or lesser extent. Throughout life the water content of connective tissue gradually diminishes, rather more so in women than in men. Concurrently, there is a decrease in the amount of amorphous material in the matrix and a relative increase in its fibrous elements.

The collagen fibres increase in thickness and develop more cross-linkages with their fellows. Where they are exposed to wear and tear they may become damaged, and their staining reactions alter; in fibrocartilage they may clump together to form what is sometimes graphically called 'asbestos'. The elastic fibres become less springy as they become thicker, and tend to fray and ultimately fragment. A decrease in their extensibility has been demonstrated.

Another important process is the deposition of calcium salts, particularly around collagen fibres; this is well seen in cartilage. As age advances, the relatively structureless matrix of hyaline cartilage is invaded by collagen fibres, so converting the tissue into fibro-cartilage; calcium is then deposited around the fibres to produce calcified cartilage, and ultimately true bone may be formed. This sort of thing begins early in adult life in the cartilages of the larynx and those which join the anterior ends of the ribs to each other and to the sternum.

The deposition of calcium in connective tissue hastens the disruption of its elastic fibres, makes it much more rigid, and increases the viscosity of the tissue hyaluronic acid. The elasticity and resilience of the tissue are thus reduced, and the loss of fluid may impede regeneration and repair, as the movement of the active cells through the tissue is necessarily hindered. In contrast to that of connective tissue, the matrix of bone loses calcium, particularly in women, and becomes porous and brittle. At the same time, the diet of many old people becomes deficient in vitamin D, and synthesis of the vitamin in the skin decreases because of lack of exposure to sunshine; their ability to absorb calcium therefore declines. This gives rise to a kind of adult rickets called osteomalacia, in which the skeleton becomes softened and may be deformed. The response to treatment with vitamin D is usually excellent. The term 'senile osteoporosis' (Fig. 11.1) describes a true condition of atrophy in which there is a quantitative reduction in the mass of bony tissue per unit volume of anatomical bone, and between youth and old age this loss may amount to about 15% of the weight of the skeleton, trabecular bone being particularly affected.

At the same time there may be a decrease in the thickness of the cortex of the long bones and the vertebral bodies, and the Haversian canals often increase in diameter and become filled with fibrous or adipose tissue.

The cause of osteoporosis is unknown, but it is more severe in women, and it appears to be the result of reduced activity of the osteoblasts. At present this is attributed to the fall in oestrogen secretion which follows the menopause;

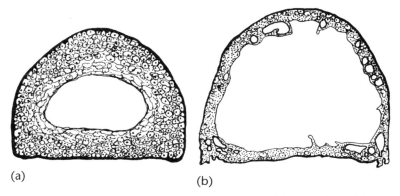

Fig. 11.1 Cross-sections of phalanges from women aged 39 (a) and 90 (b). In (b) the bone is greatly thinned, and the medullary cavity is enlarged. (Redrawn from Amprino, R., and Bairati, A. (1935). *Giorn. R. Accad. med. Torino*, **98**, 79–83.)

the level of oestrogen in the blood of men is above that of post-menopausal women. Some women may lose as much as 30% of their bone mass between the ages of 50 and 70. Other factors which have been considered as contributing to a loss of bone density include low body weight, cigarette smoking, alcohol consumption, and lack of regular exercise. Bone rarefaction of a less marked degree may simply be a feature of the normal ageing process, and attributable to an intrinsic deterioration of the performance of the osteoblasts.

Ageing of systems

Locomotor system

Because of osteoporosis, fractures are much more easily caused in elderly than in young patients, and sometimes bones may even be broken in bed as the patient tries to turn around against the resistance of the bedclothes. By the age of 80 a woman has a one in five chance of sustaining a fracture of the neck of the femur, and it has been estimated that by the age of 70 about 40% or more of women in the Western world (osteoporosis has until recently been much less common in Eastern countries such as China) will have experienced a fracture somewhere in the skeleton. Vertebrae may collapse under the load of the body weight, with resultant loss of height and pain in the back even if the spinal nerves escape damage. Unfortunately, fractures commonly do not heal properly in old people. This is in part due to the diminished mobility and multiplicative capacity of the ageing cells, although other factors are certainly involved; thus, the blood supply may be impaired, or there may be a deficiency of minerals, trace elements, or vitamins in the diet.

Osteoporosis is thus a major medical and social problem, and attempts to counter it by various means are being pursued vigorously. Calcium, fluoride, anabolic steroids, exercise, and other forms of treatment may all help, but so far the most useful treatment is hormone replacement therapy (HRT) using oestrogens and progestrogen.

Calcitonin is probably the best alternative if there is a contra-indication to oestrogen; by checking the activity of the osteoclasts, it reduces the amount of destruction.

The notochordal cells which form the fetal nucleus pulposus of the intervertebral disc begin to degenerate and die even before birth, so that by the age of about 10 years no cells are left and the nucleus is composed of white semifluid material. This is then gradually and progressively invaded by fibrous tissue from the surrounding anulus fibrosus, so that the boundary zone between the two components of the disc becomes blurred. About the age of 45–50 years, or even earlier, there is a progressive reduction in the water content of the nucleus pulposus, followed by alterations in the protein-polysaccharide complex of the nucleus, and ultimately the whole disc becomes dehydrated, pigmented, and fibrotic. At this stage it tends to collapse under strain, and this causes a decrease in height of about 3%, particularly as a result of changes in the lower part of the vertebral column, which takes the greatest gravitational load. The primary thoracic curvature, which depends mainly on the shape of the bones, is relatively little affected, but both secondary curvatures are partly undone, and the posture becomes stooping (Fig. 6.7). This is encouraged by the increasing weakness of the postural muscles which stretch across the secondary curvatures and help to maintain them. Part of this weakness may result from the distance between their origins and insertions being reduced. Similarly, the xiphisternum and ribs are brought nearer to the pubis, and the muscles of the anterior abdominal wall are slackened off. At the same time they are often required to cope with an accumulation of fat within the abdominal cavity and in the abdominal wall itself. The result is the characteristic bulging of the abdomen which occurs after middle age. Like the postural muscles of the vertebral column, the muscles of the lower limbs become weak and fail to sustain the arches of the feet. Flat feet are thus common in old age.

There have been very few longitudinal studies of adult height, but a recent cross-sectional survey in England and Wales showed that men of 60–64 years of age were about 5 cm shorter than men of 20–25. Much of this difference might be explained as a secular rather than an age effect, and the difficulties in identifying and isolating such trends by consideration of cross-sectional data have already been stressed.

Throughout the body the hyaline articular cartilages become thinner and may be eroded through, so exposing to the stresses of movement the sensitive ends of the bones rather than the insensitive cartilage. The resultant pain

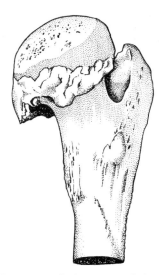

Fig. 11.2 Osteoarthritis. Showing marked erosion of the head of the femur, and out-growths of bone (exostoses) round the articular surface. (Redrawn from a specimen provided by Dr. MacCallum and illustrated in Boyd, W. (1967). *Pathology for the surgeon* (ed. Anderson, W.) 8th edn, W. B. Saunders Company, Philadelphia, by kind permission of the editor and publishers.)

makes the patient reluctant to move the joint, and this appears to encourage deposition of collagen fibres around it, so that it becomes stiff as well as painful. Bony processes known as osteophytes grow out from the margins of the articular surface and further impede movement.

The condition is known as senile osteoarthritis (Fig. 11.2), and occurs in approximately 20% of people. By the age of 60 many joints may be affected; the knee joint is the most common victim, then the acromioclavicular, the elbow, the first metatarsophalangeal, the hip, the sternoclavicular, and the shoulder joints, in order of frequency. Not only do the joints become stiff and painful, they also lose much of their stability because of the loss of tone and power in the muscles surrounding them. All three factors contribute to the cautious shuffling gait of old age.

Senile osteoarthritis is a condition which is sometimes classed as a disease, sometimes as a degeneration, and sometimes as a simple result of ageing. The loss of muscle mass and strength, as well as a concurrent reduction in maximum oxygen uptake, have profound effects in old and very old people. At 85 years of age, after a stay of 2 weeks in bed, simply dressing and undressing may lead to a maximal response of the heart rate, and getting up from a low chair or the lavatory seat may need maximal contractions of the quadriceps muscles; climbing stairs becomes an athletic feat. A survey in Sweden showed that only one healthy 79-year-old woman in three could walk fast enough across a 30 metres wide road to be fully protected by the signals at a pedestrian crossing. Much of this disability may be due to the loss of oxidative energy production by the muscle mitochondria.

The normal deterioration of the muscular system with age is aggravated by the tendency of old people to take things easy and sit at home instead of taking exercise. In 1985 a British survey found that only 9% of those aged 70 and over walked 2 miles at least once in 4 weeks.

If a limb is immobilized in plaster, the muscles under the plaster may atrophy very considerably unless exercised, particularly the quadriceps femoris, and this is a marked feature in old people. Animal work has shown that in such circumstances the loss of muscle weight results from atrophy of the individual fibres without diminution in their numbers.

Nervous system

The first manifestations of damage to the nervous system appear in the special senses; hearing is at its best at about the age of 10 years, and deteriorates thereafter. About the end of the adolescent growth spurt, reaction times begin to lengthen, particularly those involving multiple choices; the speed of simple reflexes does not alter much.

These effects are readily detectable about 20–25 years of age, and progress throughout life. The special senses also continue to deteriorate, although the effects are at first too gradual to be noticed unless accurately tested. The loss of cells is only one factor in the decline of performance. For example, the first sign of interference with vision is usually a reduction in the ability of the eye to accommodate about the age of 16, and this is probably nothing to do with loss of central control. In later life, however, functional inferiority is accompanied by anatomical evidence of cell depletion. Thus, the frequent impairment of the sense of smell is associated with atrophy of the olfactory bulb, and the inability to perceive high notes with atrophy of the nerve cells concerned. Progressive high-tone deafness is a common feature of old age, but may be the result of factors other than loss of nerve cells, such as cumulative exposure to noise, or high blood pressure.

The threshold for the taste of salt begins to increase at about the age of 20, and in those over 80 the electrical threshold for taste may be as much as five times higher than in those in their twenties. Peripheral factors are certainly involved in this case, for the number of taste buds on each circumvallate papilla drops from a figure of about 250 to about 100, and there is also a reduction in the amount of saliva secreted.

In old age there is a loss of fat in the orbits, so that the eyes become sunken, and weakness of the eye muscles affects the processes of focusing and convergence. By the age of 70, over 90% of people have some degree of opacity of the lens (senile cataract), possibly as a result of its continued growth being restrained by a tight capsule, so compressing the nucleus and the surrounding fibres, which eventually coalesce into a homogeneous mass. Another type of senile cataract results from the accumulation of fluid among the peripheral fibres, forcing them apart.

A fatty infiltration of the cornea, just inside its margin, is known as the arcus senilis, and is an almost inevitable accompaniment of old age. In one series of ophthalmic patients none over 50 was free from some degree of the condition, and in 40% of males over 60 it formed a complete and well-marked ring. It has no deleterious effect on vision, but was formerly regarded as a kind of 'marker' indicating the presence of atherosclerosis; this association is nowadays not regarded so seriously.

The macula of the retina may undergo degeneration, and senile macular degeneration is a common cause of registrable blindness.

Motor co-ordination starts to deteriorate in early adult life, and later there is some loss of control over the upright posture, so that the old person becomes unsteady and liable to fall. The autonomic system loses some of its control over bladder and bowel function, and incontinence may result; thermal regulation becomes unreliable, and there is danger from exposure to cold. The loss of cells in the substantia nigra is the cause of Parkinson's disease, in which the classical symptoms are tremor, rigidity, and slowness of movement.

In old age, the pupil may fail to dilate in darkness, and baroreflex responses may be interfered with. In about a quarter of otherwise fit elderly people the systolic blood pressure may fall by up to 20 mmHg or more when they stand up. However, it has been claimed that this condition of postural hypotension, which is one cause of the 'drop attacks' (sudden loss of consciousness resulting in falling) in old people, is due to vascular damage rather than autonomic atrophy.

Memory, and the ability to learn, are already much less efficient in early adult life than they were in childhood, and in old age short-term memory is notoriously deficient. Speech becomes slower and less assured, probably because of atrophy of the central nervous mechanisms involved. The effects of age on professionally acquired skills, apart from the decrease in physical strength, is simply a tendency towards slower, although not necessarily less accurate, working. The speed of problem solving is slowed from early adult life onwards. The changes in memory and intellectual function in what is assumed to be 'normal' old age are very similar to those of Alzheimer's disease, which may appear much earlier, perhaps at the age of 50 or less, and tends to run in families. After a few years the victim suffers confusion, disorientation, and mental and physical disability, and death occurs within 5–15 years of onset. It is associated with neurofibrillary tangles and argyrophil plaques containing amyloid protein exactly similar to those found in old age as well as in patients with Down syndrome who have reached the age of 40 or over.

It is now thought by some that these early cases of Alzheimer's disease may have a genetic basis, with a defect in a gene on chromosome 21, the same one that is affected in Down syndrome. But the whole story of this exceedingly distressing condition is very far from being elucidated. It may be that the changes in 'Alzheimer's disease' of later onset are not qualitatively different from those in normal old age, and merely differ in severity.

Recovery from nerve injuries becomes progressively less satisfactory as life lengthens. Probably the major reason for this is an inability to form new connections within the central nervous system to compensate for misdirection of nerve fibres, but an additional reason is a diminution in the ability of the damaged nerve cells to push out protoplasm to the periphery of the body.

Cardiovascular system

In the peripheral vascular system there is an increase in the tortuosity of the arteries in the hand and foot, and as early as 18 years of age those supplying the finger pads start to form a thick anastomotic network which becomes more complex with increasing age.

The walls of the arteries are a site of calcium deposition in old age, and the formerly elastic and contractile tubes may become rigid. This has important functional consequences. In the first place the vessels cannot expand in an emergency to form a collateral circulation. Secondly, there are serious effects on blood pressure. Normally, the aorta and the other elastic arteries dilate as the blood is forced into them, and their rebound maintains the diastolic pressure while the heart relaxes and the aortic valve is shut. But if the elastic arteries become relatively inexpansible the pressure in them becomes greater than normal during each cardiac contraction, but falls sharply in between. There is thus an increase in both the systolic and the pulse pressures, and a risk of haemorrhage from vessels not well supported by the adventitia or by their surroundings; for example, those in the substance of the brain.

The degenerative changes of atherosclerosis mostly affect the larger arteries, particularly at points where mechanical stresses are greatest. The plaques of fibrous and fatty material in the intima weaken the walls of the vessels, which may stretch under the increased pressure and form aneurysms. Clot is deposited on the degenerated patches, and eventually may partly or completely obliterate the lumen of the artery. Such a catastrophe quite commonly occurs in the heart, and much of the territory supplied by the affected branch of the coronary system will die and eventually be replaced, if the patient lives, by a fibrous scar.

Senile atherosclerosis is one of the characteristic degenerative changes in old age, and virtually every male over 60 years of age possesses coronary arteries in which the condition is visible to the naked eye. Females are less vulnerable, at least until after the menopause, possibly because oestrogens have a protective effect of some kind. In recent years atherosclerosis has been appearing earlier, so that it is now found in relatively young people; fatty deposits can be recognized in the wall of the aorta even in children.

The reason for this is unknown, although several factors have been proposed, among which are diet, smoking, and lack of exercise. Although none of these causes is likely in young children, a recent hypothesis proposes that infection from a micro-organism called chlamydia can lead to the build up of atheroma. Whatever is the real cause of the condition, the distinction between senescence and disease is blurred as in a number of conditions and diseases.

The heart atrophies in old age. Fibrous plaques appear in the mitral valve as early as the third decade of life; its chordae tendineae and atrioventricular ring thicken, and after about 60 calcification is common. The tricuspid valve is less severely affected, perhaps because it is subjected to less strain. The margins of the aortic and pulmonary valves become thicker and may calcify. Fat is deposited beneath the epicardium, sometimes becoming almost confluent over the whole surface of the heart, and infiltrating the walls of both atria and ventricles. Interference with the blood supply of the heart by atherosclerosis may lead to fatty degeneration of the cardiac muscle fibres.

With advancing age the sinu-atrial node loses muscle fibres, and in the atrioventricular node infiltration by fat is a feature, sometimes as early as 30 years of age. In both nodes the collagen, elastic, and reticular fibres become more prominent.

The cumulative effect of these changes is to lessen the ability of the heart to respond to demands made on it; its action becomes relatively feeble and perhaps irregular as well. The resulting poor circulation through the lungs leads to breathlessness, and the slowing down of the general circulation may lead to oedema of the feet; the toes may receive a blood supply too poor to keep them alive, resulting in senile gangrene. The venous return from the extremities is sluggish, and varicose veins either develop or become more prominent.

Haemopoietic system

Anaemia in the elderly may be due to insufficient replacement for worn-out erythrocytes. It is difficult, though, to dissociate the anaemia from the fact that some old people have a diet grossly deficient in the iron necessary for forming haemoglobin. Nevertheless, the mean haemoglobin values in an American survey of people over 84 were little different from the values of younger controls. The leucocytes of the blood diminish in number because of underproduction of lymphocytes, and the blood sedimentation rate rises.

Lymphatic system

The lymphatic system is one of the earliest to show changes. Many of its components atrophy and disappear in early adult life, especially the epitheli-olymphoid complex associated with the respiratory and digestive systems. The thymus gland is usually largely replaced by fibrous tissue before full maturity has been attained, but complete loss of thymic tissue is unusual, even in old

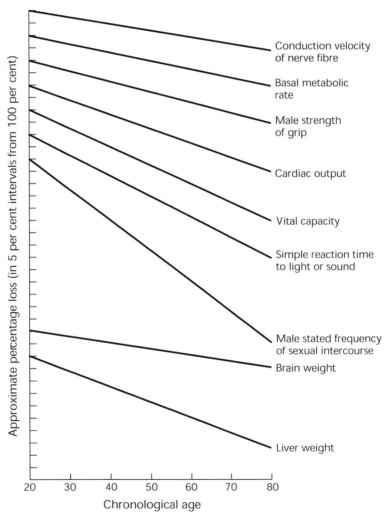

Fig. 11.3 Simplified diagram showing deterioration of various biological measurements, expressed as percentage loss of function from the ge of 20. (From Bromley, D. B. (1966). *The psychology of human aging*. Penguin books, Harmondsworth, by kind permission of the author and publishers.)

age. The structure of the lymph nodes begins to alter at puberty; the germinal centres retrogress, the cortex becomes thinner, and the distinction between cortex and medulla is less evident. In old people some nodes have a more or less uniform structure throughout. The lymphoid component of the spleen decreases around puberty, and continues to do so more gradually until old age, when the total weight of the organ falls more rapidly than the body weight.

Respiratory system

The transformation of the hyaline rib cartilages into calcified cartilage leads to inevitable interference with the mechanics of breathing. Elevation of the ribs depends largely on the ability of these cartilages to twist on themselves, thereby allowing movement between the ribs and the sternum. If this is abolished by the cartilages becoming rigid, thoracic breathing is greatly impeded (Fig. 6.2). A further problem is the obliteration, from middle age onwards, of the sternomanubrial joint, so that the sternum cannot bend on itself during inspiration, and can only move up and down as a whole, thus reducing the range of movement of the lower ribs. Movements are still further impeded by fibrosis of the joints between the upper ribs and the sternum. The rib cage falls during life, and there is loss of tone and power in the abdominal muscles and the accessory muscles of inspiration. The vertical diameter of the chest is somewhat decreased by degeneration of the thoracic intervertebral discs. All these factors interfere with breathing, and allow secretions to accumulate in the lungs.

The elasticity of the lungs themselves, which allows them to recoil during expiration, is diminished in old age, so that they do not empty themselves so efficiently, with the result that the vital capacity is reduced (Fig. 11.3). After the age of 60 the male range is 2.4–4.7l compared with 3.5–5.9l between the ages of 20 and 40. Correspondingly, the lung volume is reduced from 4.8–7.9l to 4.4–7.3l. The clinical results of these changes are shown by inefficient oxygenation, breathlessness, and liability to bronchitis, pneumonia, and fibrosis of the lung tissues.

Digestive system

In most people, some or all of the teeth have already deteriorated through disease, and may have fallen out or been removed. The gums recede, and the bone of the jaw is absorbed, leading to the angle of the mandible becoming more obtuse again; in old age it may revert to about 140°, which was the angle in the infant. The production of saliva is reduced, and the elasticity of the stomach is diminished, so that it loses its capacity to dilate following a meal.

Elderly people who retain a good appetite find this is a source of considerable dissatisfaction. In the colon there is a progressive increase in the number of diverticula, with a corresponding increase in the incidence of diverticulitis. The lumen of the appendix may be partly or completely obliterated by fusion of its walls and fibrosis; in some cases this may be the result of previous inflammation. Defecation may become disturbed because of the impaired nervous control.

The size of the liver and pancreas is reduced, and in the liver mitotic figures and binucleate cells decrease in frequency as age advances. However, regeneration occurs in senile liver just about as well as in young adults, although there is a delay in reaching the peak rate of mitosis.

Urinary and reproductive systems

The kidney becomes smaller, and after the age of about 60 the loss of kidney tissue leads to an overt impairment of excretory function, so that the blood urea tends to rise, as do the blood sugar, creatinine, and uric acid. There may be disturbances of micturition because of impaired nervous control, and very commonly difficulties are imposed upon males by enlargement of the prostate gland, which is an exception to the general rule that the weight of organs decreases in the elderly. It may become smaller at about the age of 55–60 years, but in many men this is the time when it starts to hypertrophy, and 10 years later the enlargement of the median lobe of the prostate may constitute an increasing obstruction to the passage of urine out the bladder. It is said that, after the age of 70, two in three men have some degree of urinary obstruction from this cause. In the ageing prostate the glandular component undergoes patchy atrophic change, there is a loss of the smooth muscle component relative to the connective tissue, and pigment is deposited as spheroidal granules in the smooth muscle cells. In the ducts, concretions called corpora amylacea make their appearance. The prostate also becomes increasingly likely to develop a malignant tumour within it; this particular cancer is very common in old men and often responds to hormonal treatment. Prostatic cancer in the elderly is often very slow growing and often does not cause the death of the sufferer who may well succumb as a consequence of another cause.

The seminal vesicles usually decrease in size, and yellowish pigment accumulates in their lining epithelium. There is, however, no consistent relationship between the weight of the aged prostate and that of the seminal vesicles.

Production of viable spermatozoa still continues, in at least 50% of subjects, to the age of 70 years or over; there are many examples of male fertility at ages of over 80 or even 90 years. But changes in the testicle can be detected much earlier, and consist of a reduction in size, a thickening of the basement membrane of the seminiferous tubules, a reduction in the number of interstitial cells, and an increasing fibrosis in the intertubular areas. Lipofuscin pigment is deposited in the interstitial cells and in the lining of the ductuli efferentes, and there is a gradual and considerable fall in the amount of hormone secretion in the sixth decade; this is probably responsible for many of the changes in the male sex apparatus.

The female reproductive system deteriorates in middle age. The ovaries, scarred by the escape of oocytes over the years, begin to atrophy. They may contain cysts and show other degenerative changes. Follicles cease to develop, and viable ova are not usually produced after the age of about 50 years. Because no new oocytes are formed after birth, those which are shed in the later stages of reproductive life may be 40 or more years old. This is perhaps significant in relation to the incidence of Down syndrome, which increases with increasing maternal age. After the menopause much of the ovarian stroma becomes converted into fibrous tissue, so that in old age the ovary may be represented by a mere strip of fibrosed material.

The menopause, which marks the cessation of the ovarian and uterine cycles of growth, death, and repair, occurs at a variable time in different women, but it is rare for menstruation to persist in a normal cycle much beyond the age of 50. However, just as the menarche has come to occur earlier, so the menopause appears to be occurring later in life; a century ago it seems to have been 4 or 5 years earlier than it is now, although it appears to have become stabilized for some considerable time. The age at the menopause is quite independent of the age at menarche, so that the reproductive life of different women varies in length. At the time of the menopause the quantity of oestrogens secreted by the ovaries diminishes markedly and fairly rapidly, and this affects the whole of the reproductive system. The uterus shrinks, its mucosa becomes atrophied, and the glandular tissue largely disappears. In old age it may be converted into a small fibrous mass. The vaginal epithelium thins, and there is some drying and keratinization of the vagina and vulva; the reaction of the vagina changes from acid to alkaline. Breast tissue atrophies after the menopause, probably because of the lack of ovarian stimulation, and in old age there may be little glandular tissue left, while there is a marked diminution in the fat surrounding it (Fig. 4.11). As a consequence the skin over the breast sags and wrinkles.

Endocrine system

Anatomical changes in the endocrine system have been reported, but they are often difficult to detect, and their significance is obscure. For example, it is claimed that in the adrenal medulla there is an increase in the amount of connective tissue, which forms a coarse meshwork around the parenchymal cells; there is often some dark pigment resembling melanin. In the cortex there is an increase in the number of cells containing yellow or brown pigment, and in very old people there may be conspicuous clumps of such cells. Most other endocrine glands have been said to exhibit an increasing fibrosis with age. It has been advocated that the occurrence of amyloid in the islet cells of the elderly pancreas may be a precursor of diabetes mellitus, because it is commonly found in younger people with diabetes, although, with suggestions that a virus might be involved in the causation of diabetes, this hypothesis is still unresolved.

In spite of the difficulty in finding clear histological changes in endocrine tissues, there is a well-established decline in the production of hormones by the thyroid gland, the adrenal cortex, and the gonads. The secretion of growth hormone decreases during sleep, but the plasma levels show little change; the level of gonadotrophins increases. Many older people require supplements of thyroid hormone and there is presently controversial scientific interest in the effects of giving old people supplements of growth hormone, although the effects are as yet undocumented. Testosterone levels may remain quite high but become subject to irregular fluctuations during 24 hour periods.

Skin

The main changes in the skin are a loss of subcutaneous fat, a marked diminution in the elasticity of the dermis, and a thinning of both dermis and epidermis. This thinning is difficult to measure. Figures for epidermal thickness in the antecubital fossa show an average loss of some 6 μm between the ages of 30 and 85, but some of this difference may be due to the loss of elasticity in the dermis; in youth the epidermis is 'bunched up' by the pull of the elastic fibres, and so appears to be thicker than in old age. If the epidermis is separated from the dermis before measurement, the difference in thickness with age is considerably less, but this procedure may in itself introduce other complications.

Mitosis is slowed in the germinative layer, and the viable layers of the epidermis are thinner, but the stratum corneum is more or less unchanged, and retains its main function of restricting water loss.

The deep surface of the epidermis becomes progressively smoothed; the number of dermal papillae decreases continuously after middle age, and there is a loss of the rete pegs of the epidermis. Suction blisters are thus readily produced in old skin. Measurement of the dermis is also very difficult; methods include ultrasound, the use of special callipers, and specialized radiography. The results allow it to be said that thinning progresses during adult life in males, but starts only after the fifth decade in females. The amount of collagen falls by about 1% annually throughout adult life, and fewer fibroblasts are seen in the dermis. Wrinkles are partly due to the loss of elasticity and partly to the changes in the arrangement of the bundles of collagen and of the elastic fibres in the dermis. The sagging and general loss of tension in the skin is due more to this cause than to alterations in the collagen or fluid content. The thin atrophic skin of the aged does not heal so soundly, and the sluggish blood supply tends to allow the production of ulcers. The best example of this is afforded by the 'bed-sores' that occur at the sites on which pressure is taken by the skin of bedridden people if vigorous preventive measures are not adopted. Experimental work suggests that, although the power to replace cells following a skin injury is greatest in infancy, there is little difference in the degree of cell replacement between adult and senile animals, although there is a delay in reaching the peak rate of mitosis. What is unsatisfactory is the strength of the scar; in old age collagen formation is delayed and the rate of contraction of the scar tissue is slowed. A major factor in the sometimes poor healing of wounds in the elderly is a diet deficient in both protein and vitamins.

There is a marked decline in the number of Meissner corpuscles per unit area in the dermis, and touch and vibration senses become impaired; information on other end-organs and cutaneous sensations is scanty and often contradictory.

As early as the age of 30 the replacement of terminal hairs by vellus on the vertex of the skull and in the temporal regions may become noticeable, and by 50 about 60% of males have some degree of baldness on the vertex; the number of hair follicles becomes progressively reduced with advancing age. However, there is an unexplained tendency towards increased growth of coarse hair in the nostrils and the external ears. At the same time, faulty growth processes in the remaining hairs lead to their becoming grey or white. The rate of growth of fingernails declines steadily through later life, and the nails become brittle and liable to cracking.

Theories of ageing

Since the days of Francis Bacon there has been a great deal of speculation about the possibility of finding a single 'key' cause of ageing. If such a key could be found, steps could then be taken to change the lock, and so to prolong life indefinitely. Unfortunately, things do not seem to be as simple as that, but it is perhaps worthwhile to end by discussing briefly some of the current theories regarding ageing.

Any explanation of ageing has to recognize the very strange and surprising fact that such a complex organism as the human body is unable to perform the simple tasks necessary to maintain itself in perfect condition for virtually infinity. Obviously, biology and evolution have developed so that reproduction drives the rich mix of species and the many facets of the human species and ageing, and each is therefore a key component of this process of constant change.

The process of ageing is therefore one of considerable interest to both biologists eager to understand the process and to the health professions who are faced with the problems and disease processes associated with it. Consequently, we are faced with a number of different explanations and hypotheses which attempt to explain the biology of ageing. Some of these ideas are complex and clearly beyond the remit of this text but it is worth examining some of these concepts in the context of the final stages of the life cycle.

Ageing is not a single biological process, but is in fact a series of events which can all occur at the same time at different levels within the body. For example, some changes of ageing affect the body at organ level, such as the wear and tear conditions that affect the joints, while others arise at the cell level, such as the changes that can be associated with cancers. Additionally, we must not overlook the effects of the environmental interactions and genetic variations between individuals.

There are basically four different facets of the ageing process that need to be appreciated before we look at the various hypotheses that have been developed to explain it. First, the changes associated with ageing are universal and occur in all members of the species. Secondly, ageing is intrinsic to the individual and will occur even if all environmental influences are removed. Thirdly, ageing is a progressive process, which starts slowly but gradually builds up in an accumulative fashion.

Finally, the process is bad for the organism as it results in changes that shorten life and ultimately lead to death.

The various theories of ageing fall into categories related to the biochemistry of the cellular function, to processes which are driven by genetic considerations or to theories based on the concept of accumulation of dangerous by-products within the cell.

If one examines the published literature, it rapidly becomes clear that there are many hundreds of different theories which seek to explain the biochemical basis of ageing. However, these can be classified as involving either a basic self-destruct genetic programme or a programme which is based around random chemical changes to the proteins and genes within the cell which gradually reduce its efficient working.

Programming for self destruction argues that the process of ageing is the result of a sequence of events which are already held in the programme controlled by our genes. This is a concept which is related closely to the hypothesis that development and growth is controlled by the genes. Therefore, we will expect that this genetic programme is like a time bomb, set to explode after a given time, i.e. the life-span. Genes become activated, generate ageing processes, and kill the organism. It is interesting that this approach assumes that every species of animal has a clearly defined life-span and that this process of genetic control is controlled by the nervous system and hormones in a manner similar to that of growth, development, and maturation of the younger individual. Interestingly, the evidence used to support this hypothesis comes from studies of the longevity of identical and non-identical twins where identical twins tend to have more similar life-spans than the non-identical pair.

Further support of the concept comes from work on cell culture in the laboratory, where it has been shown by a number of experiments that normal animal cells can only be propagated for a finite number of generations. This apparent inability of cells to divide for more than these predetermined numbers of generations may set a limit to the survival of tissues, which must then atrophy; if these tissues are vital ones, death must result. Hayflick described ageing as 'terminal differentiation', supposing that specific genetic systems operate to produce degenerative processes at a programmed stage in the life cycle of individual tissues and organs.

It is possible that there may be genes which assist survival in early life but act against it later; on this basis ageing results from the influence of late-acting harmful genes. This would help to explain why the harmful processes occurring in ageing have not been selected out by evolution. An investigation of very old people in Okinawa found that they had a different pattern of genes from younger controls, but it is much too early to assume that this is a basic factor in ageing.

Other theories of ageing view the constant repair of cells and their DNA as gradually becoming less efficient, leading to an accumulation of biochemical and other errors. A variation on this hypothesis suggests that cells accumulate sufficient damage to lead to destructive physiological processes which ultimately kill the cell. Extending this concept further suggests that errors arising in the DNA/RNA transfer mechanisms also are cumulative and lead eventually to a state where the cell errors are such as to lead to total catastrophe. In support of this idea is the fact that chromosomal abnormalities in human leucocytes increase from a rate of about 4% at the age of 10 years to a rate of 15% at the age of 80. There is the suggestion that the cumulative mutation in, and consequent deterioration of, the DNA of the mitochondria of cells may contribute to the phenomena of ageing and also to those of degenerative disease.

Another popular hypothesis suggests that ageing is the consequence of free radical activity. Free radicals are highly reactive molecules or atoms which can initiate chain reactions within cells and thus present a considerable hazard to all biological systems by oxidation of intracellular structures, such as the mitochondria or to proteins, and supporting tissues, such as collagen or elastin. The accumulation of these oxidized products which are resistant to the normal process of repair or turnover in the cell leads to its death. This theory is the subject of much interest as it is known that free radicals are involved in certain disease processes such as cancer, heart disease, and some diseases affecting the nervous system.

Another proposal is that the process of cell division may give rise, as a by-product, to chemicals which are necessary for the proper functioning of the daughter cells. If division becomes infrequent, cells may lose some essential component. But it has to be admitted that the potential life of a human nerve cell, on the basis of present information, is over 100 years, and there are other arguments against the hypothesis.

Certain organs, such as the ovary, have an intrinsic programmed life-span, which may depend on stimulation by the pituitary or on the number of oocytes remaining. Old ovaries transplanted into young mice are not rejuvenated, but young ovaries transplanted into old mice continue to function in their new hosts as young ovaries. Young ovaries taken from rats and stored at low temperatures can be given back to their now elderly owners and will restore oestrus.

Reproductive decline is a feature of old age in vertebrates, and attempts have been made to associate the changes of old age with the alterations in endocrine balance which occur at this time. However, the evidence so far does not support the idea that senescence is the result of a diminution in the secretion of any single hormone. The pituitary gland, in view of its close association with growth, and its known regulatory function in regard to other endocrines, is the prime suspect in such a theory, but in fact the best fit with mortality curves seems to be provided by a decline in the secretion of steroids from the adrenal cortex. Castration in either sex does not appear to shorten life (indeed, it has been claimed that eunuchs live longer than normal men) or alter the process of ageing.

The suggestion has been made that ageing in warm-blooded vertebrates might be due to their having a fixed adult size, and that the cessation of generalized growth in some way affects the power of the cells to regenerate and replace damage done by wear and tear. On this basis, animals such as the sturgeon and the large tortoises, which are supposed to remain capable of growing almost indefinitely, should not show signs of ageing. Little work has been done in this direction, but the survival curve of small fish called guppies, which also do not stop growing, does not differ very much from those of small mammals.

The blame for senescence has also been laid on the lymphatic system. Mutation in the lymphocytes, which are concerned with the immunity mechanisms of the body, might result in a steady increase in the tendency for the body to reject as foreign protein the substance of its own tissues, behaviour which is known as the autoimmune reaction.

If the Hayflick number applies in the living body, it follows that the length of life must be determined by the first vital organ to use up its quota of cell generations. Burnett suggested that the thymus gland, which is an early victim of degeneration is the most likely candidate, as it is a major factor in defending the body against mutation and degeneration.

Many people believe that the primary cause of old age is to be found in the matrix between the cells. (Alterations in the matrix might of course be a secondary result of changes in the cells which are responsible for its characteristics). Deterioration of proteins with a slow rate of replacement, such as collagen, might be involved, and the increase in the density of the matrix surrounding cells might affect diffusion through the cell membranes. It is possibly significant that in the rare condition of progeria, which has some clinical features suggestive of premature senility, there is a very striking increase in the amount of hyaluronic acid excreted in the urine.

Yet another suggestion is that the change which initiates ageing is the decline in the basal metabolic rate. So far there is little evidence for this, but the oxygen consumption of women, measured in terms of kilocalories per square metre of body surface, is 8–10% lower than that of men. This has been advanced as one reason why women tend to live longer than men because they use up energy less quickly.

The possible effects of diet, and especially diet in infancy and youth, have also aroused considerable interest due to its possible association with disease in later life. Rats fed a diet deficient in calories, but satisfactory in minerals, vitamins, and essential amino acids, remain immature for long periods. When such rats are given a normal diet they start to grow, provided that the period of deprivation has not been excessive, and may then proceed to live for up to twice as long as controls, largely because of a decrease in their liability to such illnesses as pneumonia and malignant tumours. Lesser degrees of calorie restriction, e.g. by intermittent starvation, produce proportionately lesser effects, perhaps a life-span of about $1\frac{1}{2}$ times normal. The gain in life expectancy seems to be associated with the prolongation of immaturity, as rats similarly underfed after reaching maturity show only a slight gain in life-span, which is probably attributable to the mere prevention of obesity. It is well established that rats fed a superabundant diet die sooner than controls fed a normal diet, and suffer earlier from degenerative conditions and neoplasia. There is an obvious temptation to apply these results to humans, but there are many serious obstacles. In the first place, rats have a very different growth curve. Secondly, different effects are observed in different genetic strains of rats. Thirdly, malnutrition in humans always involves deprivation of essential food materials as well as calories, and such malnutrition, whether in rats or humans, invariably shortens life. It would not be easy, and it certainly would not be ethical, to duplicate the experiments on dietary restrictions on human subjects, and until such experiments have been done there is little use speculating further.

There is no doubt that children are maturing earlier than they did formerly, and if rats live longer when they are kept immature, may not the present rapid maturation of children actually shorten their lives? It is believed that the secular trend in maturation was not a departure from normal, but rather a return to it, and such evidence as exists does not suggest that constitutional precocious puberty shortens life. Nevertheless, on a matter of such grave consequence, more information is urgently needed, and, as H. M. Sinclair has said, 'insufficient thought has been given to the most desirable rate of growth, which is not necessarily the maximum rate'. The optimal growth rate for animals has been tentatively defined by A. E. Needham as the rate which puts the least unnecessary stress on the metabolism of the animal, and he points out that few species grow at the maximum potential rate; it may therefore be a mistake to try to speed up natural growth.

It will be evident from the above that theory has far outstripped the available information, and that the prime causes of ageing are still elusive. What is needed now is an extensive programme of information gathering, and the increasing numbers of old people in the population should afford an opportunity for this. The problems of old age are inextricably mixed up with the problems of growth, and any light shed on the phenomena occurring at one end of life will immediately be relevant to investigations proceeding at the other.

From these observations, the reader will now be aware of the wide range of concepts and ideas which are being developed to explain the processes of ageing. There is little doubt about the biological outcome of the process as that is inevitably death of the organism. However, humans are social animals and with the advances in modern medicine extending the life expectancy of individuals without really having much effect on life-span, the big issue confronting societies now is not really a biological one at all but more of the social and ethical questions associated with the quality of life in the old. This issue is central to debate these days but is well beyond the remit of this text to consider.

It was Montaigne who said 'Death is but an end to dying'; it might be just as true to say that death is but an end to growing.

Further reading

Barker, D. J. P. (1994). *Mothers, babies and disease in later life.* BMJ Publishing Group, London.

Bogin, B. (1988). *Patterns of human growth.* Cambridge Studies in Biological Anthropology, Cambridge University Press.

Bromley, D. B. (1988). *Human ageing: An introduction to gerontology* (3rd edn.). Penguin Books.

Buckler, J. M. H. (1979). *A reference manual of growth and development.* Blackwell Scientific Publications, Oxford.

Buckler, J. M. H. (1994). *Growth disorders in children.* BMJ Publishing Group, London.

Bullough, W. S. (1967). *The evolution of differentiation.* Academic Press, London.

Cambell, A. G. M. and McIntosh, N. (1997). *Forfar and Arneil. Textbook of paediatrics* (4th edn.). Churchill Livingstone, Edinburgh and London.

Cameron, N. (1984). *The measurement of human growth.* Croom Helm, London.

Davies, I. (1983). *Ageing.* The Institute of Biology's Studies in Biology No. 151. Edward Arnold, London.

Eveleth, P. B. and Tanner, J. M. (1990). *Worldwide variation in human growth* (2nd edn.). Cambridge University Press, London.

Falkner, F. and Tanner, J. M. (eds.) (1986). *Human growth* (2nd edn.). Plenum Press, New York.

Blaese, R. M. (1997). *Gene therapy for cancer.* Scientific American 276 No. 6.

Greenspan, S. and Pollock, G. (eds.) (1991). *The course of life.* International Universities Press Inc., Madison, U.S.A.

Greenstein, B. (1994). *Endocrinology at a glance.* Blackwell Science, Oxford, U.K.

Greulich, W. W. and Pyle, S. I. (1959). *Radiographic atlas of skeletal development of the hand and wrist.* Stanford University Press, Stanford, Calif.

Goss, R. J. (1979). *The physiology of growth.* Academic Press, New York.

Hayflick, L. (1958). *Human cells and ageing.* Scientific American, March, 32-7.

Hauspie, R., Lindgren, G., and Falkner, F. (eds.) (1995). *Essays on auxology.* Castlemead Publications, Welwyn Garden City, U.K.

Kirkwood, T. B. (1996). *Human senescence.* BioEssays, **18**, 1009–16.

Malina, R. M. and Bouchard, C. (1991). *Growth, maturation and physical activity.* Human Kinetics Books, Champaign, Illinois, U.S.A.

Murray, A. and Hunt, T. (1993). *The cell cycle: an introduction.* Oxford University Press, Oxford.

Newman, J. (1995). *How breast milk protects new-borns.* Scientific American, December, pp. 58–61.

Reiss, M. J. (1989). *The allometry of growth and reproduction.* Cambridge University Press, Cambridge, U.K.

Roche, A. F. (1992). *Growth maturation and body composition.* Cambridge Studies in Human Biology 9. Cambridge University Press, Cambridge, U.K.

Sheldon, W. H. and Stevens, S. S. (1942). *The varieties of temperament.* Harper and Row, New York.

Sheldon, W. H. and Tucker, W. B. (1940). *The varieties of human physique.* Harper and Row, New York.

Styne, D. M. (1994). *The physiology of puberty.* Hormone Research 41, Suppl. 2, pp. 3–6.

Suzman, R. M. (1996). *The oldest old.* Oxford University Press, U.S.A.

Tanner, J. M. (1962). *Growth at adolescence* (2nd edn.). Blackwell Scientific Publications, Oxford.

Tanner, J. M. (1989). *Foetus into man* (2nd edn.). Castlemead Publication, Ware, Hertfordshire, U.K.

Tanner, J. M. and Whitehouse, R. H. (1982). *Atlas of children's growth.* Academic Press, London.

Tanner, J. M., Whitehouse, R. M., Marshall, W. A., Healy, M. J. R., and Goldstein, K. (1983). *Assessment of skeletal maturity and prediction of adult height. TW2 method.* Academic Press, London.

Thompson, D'Arcy W. (1942). *Growth and form.* Cambridge University Press, London.

Truswell, A. S. (1988). *ABC of nutrition.* British Medical Journal, London.

Ulijaszek, S. J., Johnston, F. E., and Preece, M. A. (ed.) (1998). *Cambridge Encyclopaedia of Growth.* Cambridge University Press, Cambridge, U.K.

Valman, H. B. (1989). *The first year of life.* BMJ Publishing Group, London.

Valman, H. B. (1988). *ABC of one to seven.* BMJ Publishing Group, London.

Waterston, T., Helms, P., and Ward-Platt, M. (1997). *Paediatrics: understanding child health.* Oxford University Press, Oxford, U.K.

Wilkin, T. J. (ed.) (1989). *Growth in children.* Harwood Academic Publishers, Chur, Switzerland.

Wolpert, L. (1998). *Principles of development.* Oxford University Press, Oxford, U.K.

Index